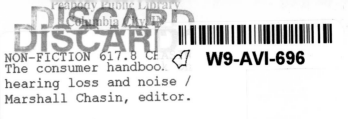

The Consumer Handbook on Hearing Loss and Noise

Marshall Chasin, Au.D., Editor

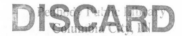

AURICLE INK PUBLISHERS
SEDONA ARIZONA

Library of Congress Cataloging-in-Publication Data
The consumer handbook on hearing loss and noise / Marshall Chasin,
editor.
    p. cm.
    Summary: "Noise interrupts sleep patterns, interferes with education
and reading, and significantly increases stress and negative emotional reactions. Writers provide various standards, present legal issues surrounding noise-induced hearing loss and subsequent tinnitus, and offer clear
strategies that can be implemented to reduce the health consequences of
noise"—Provided by publisher.
    ISBN 978-0-9825785-0-6 (hardcover)
    1. Deafness, Noise induced—Popular works. 2. Noise—Physiological
effect—Popular works. 3. Consumer education. I. Chasin, Marshall.
    RF293.5.C66 2010
    617.8—dc22

                            2009054419

First Printing
ISBN 13: 978-0-9825785-0-6
Copyright 2010

Cover concept and development by William Greaves
Concept West, Cave Creek, Arizona

This book is available at special discount rates for bulk purchases.
Contact the company for details.

Auricle Ink Publishers
P. O. Box 20607
Sedona, AZ 86341
(928) 284-0860
www.hearingproblems.com
email: AIP@hearingproblems.com

Table of Contents

Introduction i

Chapter 1 1
Hearing and Hearing Loss, Basics of Noise, and its Measurement
Marshall Chasin, AuD and Alberto Behar, PEng, CIH

Chapter 2 16
Anatomy and Physiology of the Human Ear
Richard Salvi, PhD, Edward Lobarinas, PhD and Wei Sun, PhD

Chapter 3 32
Noise: Not Just Hazardous to Your Ears–Harmful to Physical and Mental Well-Being
Arline Bronzaft, PhD

Chapter 4 49
Recreational Noise
Brian Fligor, ScD

Chapter 5 75
Why We Can't Hear in Noise
Margaret Cheesman, PhD

Chapter 6 92
Interaction between Noise and Chemicals Found in the Workplace
Thais Morata, PhD

Chapter 7 103
Tinnitus and Hyperacusis
David Baguley, PhD

Chapter 8 114
Medical Consequences of Noise
Ken Einhorn, MD

Chapter 9 129
Hearing Healthcare and the Law
Douglas A. Lewis, PhD, JD

Chapter 10 150
Standards on Occupational Noise Exposure Measurements and on Hearing Protectors
Alberto Behar PEng, CIH and Lee Hager

Chapter 11 163
Architectural Strategies to Minimize Noise
William J. Gastmeier, MASc PEng

Glossary 181

Index 196

Introduction

Only three things are certain in life, death, taxes, and age-related hearing loss. It would be nice to do away with the first and second, but realistically all we can do is minimize the third. Hearing loss affects everyone and in most cases, is very slow in its progression. And because it is so slow and gradual, people generally do not recognize hearing loss for what it is. They may gradually withdraw from many noisy social situations and in some cases, stop interacting socially. It's understandable that friends and family may notice this long before an individual does. A person with a hearing loss might comment that speech is mumbled or may say, "I can hear you fine; it's just that you're mumbling." A family member would say, "Uncle Frank is becoming very quiet and antisocial."

These situations are not unusual. The two most common causes of hearing loss are presbycusis (hearing loss associated with aging) and noise exposure. While being over the age of 75 is not preventable, hearing loss from MP3 players or construction sites can be prevented. There are many things that can be done to prevent many forms of hearing loss. The question therefore becomes, "What can be done today to prevent hearing loss tomorrow?"

The ear is an amazingly complex organ and it always surprises me to see what is going on in the space no larger than the tip of your small finger. This book is written for the consumer—those of you who have some hearing loss and those who don't want to lose more hearing. As you may already know, noise can interrupt sleep patterns, but it can also interfere with education and reading, and increase stress levels. Many chapters have clear strategies that can be implemented to reduce these challenges. You might find it helpful to know the reasons why you cannot hear in noisy environments as well as in quiet locations and learn strategies to improve communication in noise. We cover the insidious effects of, and some of the explanations behind tinnitus (ringing in the ears) and an associated problem of a reduced tolerance for loud sounds. Architectural designs and the strategies to minimize residential and office noise are covered. Some pharmaceuticals can be used to minimize the effects of noise by "mopping up" certain chemical compounds that may be implicated in hearing loss. They'll be discussed as well as listening to the advice of an otolaryngologist who examines the health consequences of noise. There are various standards that have been implemented to minimize the effects of noise on hearing and well-being

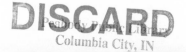

that you may want to know. There are also legal issues surrounding noise-induced hearing loss presented by a dual-licensed practitioner—an audiologist and a lawyer.

I recommend that you approach this book as you would any helpful handbook—take from it everything you can that will benefit you to enhance your quality of life. Preview the Table of Contents and look for the chapters that most apply to your issues. Peruse the Index in the back of the book looking for catchwords and phrases that cover topics of interest to you. Take advantage of the detailed Glossary in the back of the book that defines terms in case as you read you forget their meaning. This book is not intended as a John Grisham novel. It may not be necessary for you to read all chapters. Nevertheless, we authors have gathered to help educate you in the broadest ways possible where you might need information. So go for it. Wear out the pages!

I would like to thank the many contributors in this book. These authors comprise some of the world's most well-respected researchers and professionals and I wish to thank them for their time, their passion, and their commitment to the moderation of the effects of noise on our bodies, minds, and ears.

Enjoy!

Marshall Chasin, Au.D.
Editor

The Consumer Handbook

on

Hearing Loss and Noise

CHAPTER ONE

Hearing and Hearing Loss: Basics of Noise and its Measurement

*Marshall Chasin, Au.D., M.Sc., Aud(C), Reg. CASLPO
and Alberto Behar, P.Eng., CIH*

Dr. Chasin is an audiologist and the Director of Auditory Research at the Musicians' Clinics of Canada. He is also the Coordinator of Research at the Canadian Hearing Society, Adjunct Professor at the University of Toronto (in Linguistics) and an Associate Professor in Audiology at the University of Western Ontario. Dr. Chasin received his B.Sc. in mathematics and linguistics at the University of Toronto, a M.Sc. in Audiology and Speech Sciences at the University of British Columbia, and his Doctor of Audiology (Au.D.) degree from the Arizona School of Health Sciences. He serves on the board of several hearing loss prevention organizations such as Hearing, Education, and Awareness for Rockers (HEAR) and the Association of Adult Musicians with Hearing Loss (AAMHL). He has also served as the editor or a member of the editorial board of several industry and scholarly peer reviewed publications. He has served on several governmental and regulatory committees, both at the local and the national level. Dr. Chasin has been involved with hearing and hearing aid assessment since 1981 and is the author of over 200 clinically based articles. He has lectured extensively, and is the author or editor of several books.

Alberto Behar is a Professional Engineer and Certified Industrial Hygienist. He holds a Diploma in Acoustics from the Imperial College (London, UK, 1971) and has been the recipient of several Fellowships, including one from the Fulbright Commission (USA) and the Hugh Nelson Award of Excellence in Industrial Hygiene (OHAO, Canada). Since 1990, he has been the President of Noise Control and Management consulting company dealing with occupational and environmental noise and vibration as well as with hearing conservation and protection, fields he has been active in for over 40 years. He is Research Associate with the Sensory Communication Group, IBBME, (University of Toronto) and since 2004 Adjunct Assistant Professor at the Department of Public Health Sciences, University of Toronto. Alberto is a chairman and member of CSA and ANSI committees and working groups and is also the Canadian representative at two ISO Working Groups.

Introduction

Sound is a marvelous energy. It can convey signals that warn like a horn, or that bring great joy or comfort like gentle words spoken from the heart. *Sound* is a vibration in any elastic medium (such as through air, water or steel). The beauty of sound is both in its simplicity and complexity. The simplest sound is a pure tone single frequency sine wave (~). Its complexity evolves when many sounds are mixed together, like the image on the cover of this book, or like the blending of many musical instruments in an orchestra. The instruments generate a magnificent array of frequencies that bring great pleasure to our ears, from subtle tones to loud crescendos. Conversely, imagine that an entire orchestra played completely off key. This would resonate through our ears and be perceived in our brains as a terrible *noise* (defined as unwanted sound), perhaps no different from a screen door in the wind banging against the house. It's all *noise*.

Sound travels through air at 1,125 feet a second (which equates to about 768 miles an hour). In water it travels at approximately 4,400 feet a second depending on the water temperature (for example, 4,700 feet a second if the water temperature is 59° F). In the Old West, remember the movies where a character put his ear to the railroad track? He could hear the vibration of the train coming (16,000 feet a second in steel) long before he could see it or hear the sound traveling through air.

Noise is always sound, but sound is not always noise. Noise is a subjective interpretation of sound. Sound comes from many different sources and is comprised of many different elements, most of it adding richness to life, like speech and music. However, noise has progressively become a part of our lives in ways we would often like to avoid. Typically, noise carries no information. That is, there's nothing meaningful about it. This helps to distinguish it from speech and music, yet really doesn't explain why noise can be so bothersome and most forms of music are pleasant. For most of us, the sound of a rattle in the car is noise. A neighbor's barking dog is noise. The racket of a cocktail party if you're not part of it is noise. These are "random phase" events, a fancy way of saying there's nothing meaningful about the vibration. When scientists at SETI (Search for Extraterrestrial Intelligence) aim their radio signal dishes up into the sky, they're receiving many random phase signals that they ignore. In fact, a non-random signal might cause alarms to go off!

This characteristic of noise (random phase) allows us to focus on speech or music in the presence of background noise. We will leave the specifics about how this is accomplished to later chapters, but suffice it to say that the human brain is an amazing computer that allows us to understand speech in the presence of noise—to a point. We've all been in a noisy social gathering and regardless of our hearing ability, just could not distinguish what was being said. Now let's turn to the receivers of the noise—our ears and brain—and the process of how we hear and interpret sound.

Hearing and Hearing Loss

You've just scheduled your first appointment to see an audiologist in order to check your hearing. You have no major concerns, but perhaps because you're over 50, your family physician has suggested that this would be a good idea. The first thing the audiologist does is take your case history. This involves questions about noise exposure, including occupational, military exposure, and recreational noise such as hunting or the use of MP3 players. A family history is also taken including the hearing status of your siblings and parents in order to determine any familial or genetic connection, as well as any ear-related operations. Questions are also asked concerning ear-related non-hearing elements (such as balance issues), and head noises such as tinnitus (ringing or buzzing in the ear). Finally, any good history would be "interactive" with the hopes that you are able to fill in any blanks about your hearing or communication problems that were not asked.

You and the audiologist will now take a short stroll into the next room where there's a sound-treated booth for the actual hearing test. These specially designed booths essentially eliminate all extraneous noise. The "hearing test" actually comprises a number of tests that when taken together, with the history, give a good picture of your hearing status.

It usually starts with "pure tone" audiometry. A set of specially calibrated earphones are used to present a series of beeps or tones. You're instructed to indicate when you hear the tones, even if they're very faint. In this way, the softest level at which you can hear the tones is established. This is referred to as *threshold*, and is done for octave frequencies 250-8000 Hz. *Frequency* is the number of vibrations (cycles per second) in a sound wave, also referred to as "Hz" (pronounced *hurts,* named after the famous German physicist

Heinrich Hertz who discovered the existence of radio waves). You might be more familiar with the term *pitch*, which is the psychological counterpart to frequency, and essentially means the same thing. The ear and brain interpret frequency as *pitch*.

The low frequency end of the scale at 250 Hz is very close to middle C on the piano. Notes that are below middle C are typically not assessed since there's very little speech energy that low. Also, it becomes rather difficult to say whether you "heard" or "felt" the sound at very low frequencies. Vowels typically have a lot of their energy around 250 Hz. Consonant energy is in the higher frequencies, around 2k-4k Hz. This comprises many of the "hissing" sibilant-type consonant sounds, such as /s/, /sh/, or /f/. The hearing thresholds for these low and high frequencies are graphed on a chart known as an *audiogram.* Figure 1-1 shows an audiogram for a person with normal hearing for most of the vowels in speech, but with reduced hearing sensitivity for some of the higher frequency consonant sounds. Since most of the clarity (intelligibility) for speech is derived from higher frequency consonant sounds, the person represented here might say, "I hear you, but I don't understand you." That is, the low frequency vowels sounds are quite audible, but the important consonant sounds that carry the clarity in speech are not heard or are distorted.

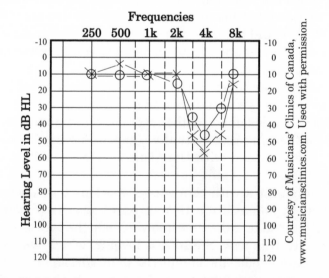

Figure 1-1: Audiogram shows hearing threshold results ("O" for the right ear and "X" for the left ear) with a typical noise-induced hearing loss worse in the 4000 Hz region

The next aspect of the hearing test involves word recognition testing. A list of 25 or 50 single syllable words are given to the person either live-voice or recorded. Anyone with normal hearing is expected to correctly repeat 92-100% of the words (e.g., "ball," "fire," "chair"). Lower scores are most commonly found in people with more significant hearing loss. For example, someone with a severe hearing loss might only understand 50% of speech; that is, they'd only understand about half of what is said in a conversation.

The thresholds recorded on the audiogram by a professional should be reliable, and periodic assessments will show if there's been a change in hearing. We know that under test conditions as the ability to hear higher frequency tones decreases, the ability to understand in noise also decreases in the real world. To add to the diagnostic complexity, two people with the same audiogram may function quite differently in a quiet or noisy environment. This is in part related to how our brains receive and ultimately interpret sounds. Our ability to hear in noise is as much a brain issue as an ear issue. This distinction may help explain why some people are more bothered than other people by everyday noise in our environment.

Conductive and Sensorineural Hearing Loss

A detailed explanation of hearing loss is found in chapter 2, but an overview here is worthwhile. Hearing loss can occur in the outer (ear canal) or middle ear (area containing an air space, three tiny bones and the Eustachean tube). These conditions are usually temporary and can be medically or surgically treated. The middle ear is the portion commonly subject to ear infections and the effects of pressure changes (like when your ears pop during altitude changes). Hearing loss in either the outer or middle ear is known as *conductive* because the conduction or transmission of sound to the sense organ (inner ear) is blocked. A person with a conductive type hearing loss would hear things weakly but clearly, and if the volume was turned up, would hear well without straining. It's analogous to listening to a radio with the volume turned down. Turning up the volume resolves the difficulty. Examples of some causes of conductive hearing loss include wax impaction, middle ear fluid, a perforation of the eardrum, and a stiffening of the middle ear bone (otosclerosis).

Hearing loss that is related to the inner ear (cochlea) is typically permanent and usually cannot be restored by medical, surgical, or other means. This type of hearing loss is known as *sensorineural* and is analogous to having the radio tuned slightly off-station. Regardless of the volume setting on the radio, it'll never be as clear as for someone who has a conductive hearing loss. Examples of some causes of a sensorineural hearing loss include presbycusis (associated with aging), occupational noise exposure, recreational noise exposure, certain medications, viruses, and congenital problems (hearing loss from birth). We refer to it as sensorineural because it could be sensory (hair cell damage in the inner ear), neural (damage to the hearing nerve that brings auditory impulses to and from the brain) or both. Audiological tests are specifically designed to differentiate the various kinds of hearing loss. One reason why two people can function differently in a noisy environment despite having similar audiograms is that one person may have more neural involvement than the other. Generally, those with more of a neural component will function more poorly than those with a purely sensory problem.

The Decibel

On the audiogram in Figure 1-1 we see that frequency, measured in Hz, is written across the top. Down the side of the audiogram is a measure of hearing loss in decibels (written as dB). It will be helpful if you refer to this as we discuss the decibel scale, and if you have a copy of your own audiogram, you may better understand its interpretation as we move along.

A decibel is a unit of sound pressure. It's a measure like temperature in the sense that there is a 0 degree mark and everything is measured relative to that. When someone tells you it's zero degrees Fahrenheit outside, you understand exactly what that means. The corresponding 0 dB on a decibel scale is not the absence of sound, any more than 0° F is the absence of temperature; albeit, 0 dB is very soft and has to have a known reference to have meaning.

Hearing Level (HL or HTL)

On an audiogram, "dB HL" means hearing level as measured in decibels. The corresponding suffix "HL" following the acronym dB defines what the 0 dB reference is, just like the suffix in temperature. For example, 30° is meaningless unless we know what reference scale is used, such as Fahrenheit or Celsius (30° F is quite different from 30° C!). In the case of hearing measurement, 0 dB HL was standardized on the hearing of thousands of young adults who had no history of ear problems or noise exposure. The 0 dB point was the lowest level at which this group could hear various tones 50% of the time. The last such survey was performed in the late 1960s (ANSI S3.6-1969) and all audiometers need to be calibrated annually to this standard. This ensures that the obtained thresholds are consistent from audiometer to audiometer. Some audiograms such as that seen in Figure 1-1 use dB "HTL" (Hearing Threshold Level) which means the same thing as HL.

Sound Pressure Level (SPL)

In the area of risk management for noise (and many other scientific areas) another type of reference point for decibels is used—Sound Pressure Level (SPL). Its zero reference is .0002 dynes per cm² and was chosen because it's relatively close to the quietest sound that we can hear. Also, in the 1920s when the SPL scale was first standardized, 0 dB SPL was easy to measure with the technology of the time. Inexpensive commercially available sound level meters (such as the one shown in Figure 1-2) can be purchased for less than $100 and can measure the noise level in dB SPL. However, inexpensive sound level meters cannot accurately measure sound levels below 40 dB SPL.

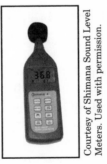

Courtesy of Shimana Sound Level Meters. Used with permission.

Figure 1-2: Sound level meter that can measure sound on a variety of decibel scales

These devices provide a reading directly in dB, so the measurement is easy to obtain and there's no need for calculations. Most sound level meters can display noise levels as dBC or dBA. The dBC (no filtering) scale is also known as *linear*. However, it's seldom used for measuring sound levels related to human hearing and is not relevant to this discussion. The dBA scale uses an electronic circuit that filters out some low frequency sounds in order to mimic the sensitivity of the human ear. It is the dBA scale that functions as a simulation of the sounds that actually can reach the human inner ear, and for this reason, is our focus.

This is very useful for measuring the levels of noise and music, since the human auditory system seems to become damaged in well-defined ways by an excessive level of noise measured on the dBA scale. The A filter provides different attenuations at different frequencies. This scale is based on the dB SPL scale, but further modified to "simulate" human hearing by filtering (taking away) well-defined amounts of sound in the low frequency range. The filter is set at 0 dB at 1000 Hz, 9 dB at 500 Hz, 15 dB at 250 Hz, and so on. This filter is used because the human outer and middle ear collects, directs and amplifies sound going into the inner ear, and alters sound pressure for the lower frequencies. Therefore, what ultimately gets through is quieter for lower frequency sounds (comparable to the left side of the piano keyboard) than higher frequency sounds. The human ear is a wonderfully complex mechanism, but it does fall short on its ability to handle sounds in the lower frequencies. In a way this may be a good thing because much of the intrusive low frequency industrial noise never gets through to the inner ear. The result is less potential risk of damage than if we had a broader spectrum hearing system.

The person whose audiogram is shown in Figure 1-1 suffered from the result of long-term noise exposure. This is actually the audiogram of a rock and roll drummer, but similar types of hearing loss are found in cases of occupational and military noise exposure. The important question here is what is the sound level that can potentially be damaging to the inner ear mechanism? That number turns out to be 85 dB on the A scale (85 dBA) or higher, if exposed for a whole working day. This is the result of many decades of research, but like all things in life, this one number doesn't tell the entire story.

We know from industry and research that 85 dBA for 40 hours a week will eventually result in a permanent sensorineural hearing loss. The greater the sound level and/or the longer the duration of exposure, the greater will be the hearing loss. For example, 85 dBA for 40 hours a week poses the same risk criteria for exposure to 88 dBA for only 20 hours a week, 91 dBA for only 10 hours a week, and so on. For each increase of 3 dB, the potential damage is approximately doubled. Stated differently, for each 3 dB increase, one can only be exposed for half the time in order to have the same risk (potential damage). Table 1-1 shows this relationship. The 3 dB figure is frequently referred as the "3 dB exchange rate," meaning that a 3 dB increase in sound level can be "exchanged" for cutting the duration of exposure in half. In light of current knowledge and understanding of risk criteria, most people should be able to enjoy without hearing loss a concert that does not exceed 95 dBA so long as exposure does not exceed 4 hours (and they don't do anything too noisy for the rest of the week). As will be discussed in later chapters, many city noise regulations are based on the figure 85 dBA and the 3 dB exchange rate.

Sound Levels (dB A)	Duration of Exposure (hours)
85	40
88	20
91	10
94	5
97	2.5
100	75 minutes
103	37.5 minutes

Table 1-1: Various sound levels in dBA reading for a specified duration all yield the same exposure level

Where the 3 dB Exchange Rate Breaks Down

There are two main ways that the inner ear can be permanently damaged from noise exposure. One is related to long-term exposure at a level and duration that exceeds the numbers found in Table 1-1. This type of hearing loss is gradual and may take years to notice. In many cases a person may observe that people are starting to mumble (especially in noisier social situations) or find that they suffer from ringing in the ears or head (known as *tinnitus*—pronounced tih-NEYE'-tuhs or TIHN'-ih-tuhs). People may slowly withdraw from social interaction simply because they can no longer understand speech clearly, and they may not realize it's related to hearing loss. If the noise level is up to about 115 dBA (extremely loud), the 3 dB exchange rate rule works, but notice from Table 1-1 that even at 110 dBA, the maximum duration would be less than 10 minutes a week. Managing the safety to exposures above 115 dBA cannot be predicted with any degree of certainty and should be avoided at any cost. The second way that the inner ear can be permanently damaged from noise is from acoustic trauma. As the name suggests, extremely intense sound can cause a sudden and permanent hearing loss even if the duration is brief. This is, in most cases, related to an explosive sound such as gunfire, fireworks, eruption of a pressure valve, chemical explosions, and so forth.

The physiologies of these two mechanisms are quite different. The first is lower intensity long-term exposure, causing a gradual wearing down of thousands of nerve fibers (hair cells) in the inner ear; the second is acoustic trauma, a "ripping out" of the nerve endings and their supporting structures as the result of a single acoustic event. Both ultimately result in hearing loss that is not medically treatable, and will be discussed further in Chapter 2. The main rehabilitative approaches include hearing aids, assistive technologies (for example, amplified telephones and television), and aural rehabilitation (hearing management classes that include lipreading and provide a better understanding of hearing loss through group interaction with an instructor).

It has recently been discovered that certain pharmaceutical drugs can reduce the damage to the ear caused by loud noise and this has to do with altering the metabolic byproducts of cells. When a person is subjected to loud noise the metabolism of the cells in the inner ear increase and generate a form of oxygen that contains free radicals. This can be quite toxic to the structures of the inner ear. One strategy that appears to offer some relief is use of antioxidants that serve to mop up the toxic oxygen molecules and thereby preserve hearing. (Many food sources are rich in antioxidants including blueberries, cranberries, pinto beans and red kidney beans.)

In some research studies using animals, the antioxidant is injected directly into the inner ear. However, this is not clinically feasible. Other research has looked at antioxidant medication taken orally which is then absorbed by the entire body, in hopes that some of it will find its way to the inner ear. One such antioxidant is called L-*N*-acetyl-L-cystine, or more simply "L-NAC" and may be found as an ingredient in over-the-counter supplements sold in health food stores. Early results of an oral antioxidant (such as L-NAC) appear quite promising; however, it should not be considered a cure for inner ear hearing loss or used in lieu of hearing protection or in conjunction with other methods in the belief that this will minimize the risks of exposure to loud noise.

There are a few other pharmaceutical routes being investigated, such as medications that prevent inner ear cell death from loud noise; however, this research is still in the early phases and none of these have received approval from the Food and Drug Administration (FDA)

Lower Levels of Noise Exposure

There's a small (but measurable) permanent sensorineural hearing loss *that can occur* from long-term exposure to levels between 80-85 dBA. This does vary from person to person, and the permanent hearing loss is so small that it would not typically be noticed by the individual. This is why most local ordinances establish 85 dBA and not 80 dBA as their upper limit. However, the effects of long-term noise exposure from intensities less than 85 dBA can cause measurable hearing loss. Depending on the study, permanent hearing loss between 5 and 9 dB will occur at 4000 Hz for long-term exposure to noise at 85 dBA. So 85 dBA is not exactly safe, but for all intents and purposes, it's a number that regulators and factory operators want to achieve in order to protect their workers. There's also research that indicates that exposure levels below 85 dBA can be even more damaging if the worker is also exposed to certain toxic chemicals that may be found in the workplace.

Chapter 3 has been dedicated to this issue since difficulties resulting from noise are not just restricted to hearing loss. As will be seen, noise levels that are lower than 85 dB have been implicated in studies of sleep disruption, work interference, increased stress, and delayed cognitive and educational development as evidenced by lower reading scores among students. Cases of increased fetal heart rates in pregnant women have also been linked to long duration lower-level noise exposure.

The Basics of Sound

At this point you may be wondering if this is a textbook! It isn't. We merely have to define and discuss sound, noise, frequencies, decibels, SPLs and the like because a fundamental working knowledge is important to better understanding the information that will follow in other chapters.

To propagate sound, there is a need for two elements. One is a vibrating surface, like the wall of a bell, a musical instrument or the vocal cords of a speaker. The other, as important as the first, is an elastic medium that transmits the sound to the surrounding world.

Let's explain this concept a bit better by taking you on a mythical trip. Pretend for the moment that we're all immersed in the Ocean of Air that is made up of an immense number of molecules. We can picture those molecules as small balls that bounce one against the other in a completely random way without any order or predictability. As long as the ambient temperature is above absolute zero (-273^0C) which is slightly colder than that found in outer space, we do have this kind of random motion (also known as *Brownian motion*).

Now, what happens to the molecules that are surrounding our vibrating surface? Those little balls get "organized." That is, they follow the motion of the surface, going back and forth, and in turn, push other adjacent molecules that are not in contact with the surface, but are subjected to the same motion transmitted from the former surface "balls." This is called *propagation*: a phenomenon by which the motion of the original vibrating surface "travels" as a wave in all directions provided there is a medium (in this case air). We can't have sound without a medium within which the balls/molecules can move. Sounds cannot be propagated in a vacuum.

So now we have sound traveling from the source in all directions at the speed of approximately 1,125 feet per second (or about a fifth of a mile per second, depending on air pressure) thanks to the motion of the molecules that bounce into one another. In a thunderstorm, if thunder is heard about 5 seconds after a lightening flash, then the lightening was about 1 mile away. Now, what happens when the sound meets a body, such as a wall, a person or an eardrum? Obviously, the last molecule that reaches the surface will stop dead, since it cannot penetrate a solid object. And here, we have this little molecule "pushing" the wall; exerting force against the surface.

In physics, pressure is defined as the relation of force divided by the surface to which it is applied. In this case, because it's caused by sound, we call this pressure *sound pressure*. It's directly related to the force of the sound (louder sound equals larger sound pressure).

With respect to human hearing sensitivity, being able to hear pressure changes created by the smallest movement of molecules represents an incredible ability to hear. This pressure can be measured at its lowest and highest impact on human hearing, from the softest sound we can hear to our threshold of pain. This comprises a range of 1,000,000 between the faintest noise that we can perceive and the one that will cause pain to our ears. The decibel (dB) scale helps us manage this extraordinary range. Using dB, the range of sound pressure level (SPL) is reduced from 1,000,000 to 1, to a range of 120 to 1, something much easier to manage. For example, the numbers 10 and 10,000 are quite different, but the logarithmic equivalents are 1 and 4 respectively—again a much more manageable range. Table 1-2 shows examples of SPLs that we may find in everyday life.

Common Household Items	Sound Levels (dBA)
Blender	83
Hair dryer (at ear)	91
Vacuum cleaner	80
Lawn mower	94
MP3 player (volume 8/10)	96

Table 1-2: Some common household items and their approximate sound level in dBA

Because decibels are logarithmic expressions, the dB cannot be added directly (the pressures can but not the decibels). In other words, if a machine generates a sound level of 90 dB SPL and we place another one also generating 90 dB SPL in close proximity, the resulting sound level is not 180 dB, but 93 dB.

Of interest here is that 93 dB SPL is twice the sound pressure as 90 dB SPL, so it's potentially twice as damaging. Yet, the perceived change in loudness from this 3 dB increase may be barely noticeable. Humans are great at discerning small differences in frequency (we can easily tell if a singer is off key) but we're more challenged in discerning small differences in sound pressure.

The Occupational Safety and Health Administration (OSHA)

The Occupational Safety and Health Administration (OSHA: www.osha.gov) sets the rules about safe noise levels for US companies and employees, but has no enforcement or regulatory control. That is left up to each state. OSHA has established the guidelines for the two risk factors surrounding hearing loss and noise: the level of noise, and the duration of exposure. But another factor that must be understood is the noise exposure level. This is a measure of the combination of both of these two factors. The noise exposure level is indicated as L_{eq} (pronounced "L.E.Q.") and is the level of a steady sound whose level is equivalent to the measured one from the point of view of its effects on the hearing of the exposed person. L_{eq} is based on a 3 dB exchange rate meaning that the effect of increasing (or decreasing) of the noise level is the same, provided the exposure time is decreased (or increased) <u>two times</u>. As an example, an 8 hr exposure at 85 dBA is equivalent to a 4 hr exposure to 85 + 3 = 88 dBA.

However, for the time being, OSHA requires an exchange rate of 5 dB. The noise exposure level using 5 dB exchange rate is known as L_{OSHA}. It is expected that the Environmental Protection Agency (EPA) will adopt in the near future the use of the L_{eq}, as is done in most other countries. There's no scientific evidence to support the 5 dB exchange rate. It was merely an administrative decision made by OSHA many years ago. As per L_{OSHA} in the above example, an 8 hr exposure at 85 dBA is equivalent to a 4 hr exposure to 85 + 5 = 90 dBA.

Personal Noise Exposure Measurement

A noise dosimeter is worn by a person at risk who is concerned about the possibility of losing hearing based on the level of a specific noise exposure. It is a specialized sound level meter that specifically measures noise exposure (in dBA) over time and integrates the total exposures so that the result is representative of the risk. At the end of the measurement period, the instrument shows the noise exposure as L_{eq} or L_{OSHA}, depending on how it's set up. Many dosimeters allow for the simultaneous measurement of both magnitudes. A noise dosimeter also measures "dose" with 100% being the maximum recommended (e.g., 85 dBA for 40 hours a week). Figure 1-3 shows a consumer dosimeter that can be worn all day. It provides information on the percentage dose to which wearers have subjected themselves. Anything in excess of 100% can be problematic and special measures should be taken to reduce it, such as the use of hearing protection and/or removing the worker from the noisy environment.

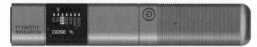

Photo courtesy of Etymotic Research, Inc. Used with permission.

Figure 1-3: Dosimeter that can clip onto a shirt that gives results in terms of percentage of dose

Figure 1-4 shows a pictorial audiogram representing a variety of common noise exposures, their frequencies, and sound levels. As you can note, it doesn't take much to reach dangerous sound levels.

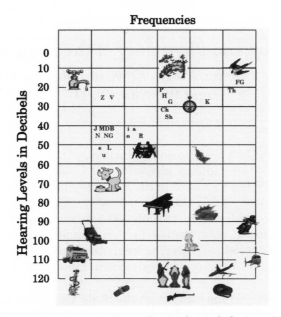

Frequencies

Figure 1-4: Pictorial representation of sounds and their noise levels

Conclusions

As you've learned, among the many causes of preventable hearing loss, noise exposure is number one. From city to city and country to country, we share a common problem. Noise has become an invasive, unwelcome partner in all industrialized nations. According to the World Health Organization (WHO), one in five Europeans is regularly exposed to sound levels at night that could have a significant impact on health. Research at the University of Melbourne (Australia) has revealed that city noise is now interfering with the mating croak of frogs. But it's not just frogs at risk. A 2009 WHO publication provides evidence of the damage night noise can do to people's health and offers guidelines for sound levels at night in Europe. The European Environmental Agency announced in late 2009 that 67 million city residents living in communities larger than 250,000 people endure noise levels of 55 dB or more, continuing into the night. Their concern now is the failing health of residents exposed to these "hazardous" noise levels in the city—Paris, France named the noisiest.

As you've read, prolonged exposure to sounds exceeding 85 dBA will eventually cause permanent hearing loss. The potential damage increases as a function of increasing sound levels. As you'll read in Chapter 3, these risks hold very serious health consequences.

CHAPTER TWO
Anatomy and Physiology of the Human Ear
Richard J. Salvi, Ph.D., Edward Lobarinas, Ph.D. and Wei Sun, Ph.D.

Dr. Salvi has a Ph.D. in Experimental Psychology from Syracuse University and did a post-doc in auditory physiology at Upstate Medical Center in Syracuse. Dr. Salvi is a Professor in the Department of Communication Disorders and Sciences and is the Director of the Center for Hearing and Deafness. He has published more than 300 papers related to anatomy and physiology of hearing, otoacoustic emissions, auditory plasticity, hair cell regeneration, noise-induced hearing loss, ototoxicity, age-related hearing loss, tinnitus and brain imaging of tinnitus in humans and animals.

Dr. Lobarinas received his Ph.D. from the State University of New York at Buffalo. Currently, he holds a Research Assistant Professor appointment at the Center for Hearing and Deafness and is a clinical Audiologist. Originally trained in Behavior Pharmacology at Rutgers University where he did his undergraduate education, he has focused his research on finding treatments for tinnitus using animal models. Dr. Lobarinas developed his own animal model of tinnitus and has continued to explore novel treatments for tinnitus as well as using objective measures such as brain imaging to find neural correlates of tinnitus.

Dr. Sun is Assistant Professor in the Department of Communicative Disorders and Sciences at the State University of New York at Buffalo. He was trained as an electrical engineer and then obtained his Ph.D. in audiology in the State University of New York at Buffalo. He has broad research interests including cellular physiology of spiral ganglion neurons, developmental change in the central auditory system affected by environmental noise and neonatal nicotine exposure, and the central auditory system reorganization related to tinnitus and hyperacusis. Dr. Sun's research projects are funded by NIH, the Royal National Institute for Deaf People and the American Federation for Aging Research.

Whether we listen to music, speech, or noise, the sound waves that enter the outer ear are transmitted to the middle ear and are "sensed" in the inner ear. From here, sound, which is now in the form of electrical impulses travels by the auditory nerve into the hearing regions of the brain where neurological and biochemical processes allow us to "hear" the sound. This chapter will review some of the important features of our hearing mechanism that play an important role in perceiving the pitch and loudness of sound. For this, we need to discuss four parts of the ear—the external ear, middle ear, inner ear or cochlea, and the central auditory pathway.

The External Ear

The only visible part of the auditory pathway is the external (outer) ear. This is the part of the head where we hang our glasses and is a crescent-shaped structure. It's composed of cartilage that gives it shape as well as flexibility. When one looks at the outer ear there are a series of characteristic contours of nooks and crannies as well as a bowl (the concha) leading to the opening of the canal. Like all chambers, the tubular opening with its nooks and crannies have *resonant frequencies* (the number of cycles per second at which a mass vibrates most easily), like what is heard when you blow across the top of a pop bottle. By placing a small microphone in the ear canal, these resonant frequencies can be measured. The cartilage that forms the nooks and crannies adds to the stability of the outer ear so it won't flop over. The resonant frequencies are just along for the ride—they are inherent side effects of having all these "nooks and crannies." The concha has a resonant frequency consistent with its size and shape—around 4500 Hz—the high-pitched area where many important speech consonants are. It's possible that this concha bowl in the outer ear serves to pre-emphasize the loudness of /s/ and /th/ before they even reach the sense organ (cochlea) of the ear. Another possible use of the concha bowl is resonance that gives us localization cues in the vertical plane. For example, it helps to identify from where sound is coming from if it is slightly above us.[1] Finally, a one-inch long tube known as the *external auditory meatus* (ear canal) extends inwardly from the concha and terminates at a thin coned-shaped sheet of tissue called the *tympanic membrane* (eardrum).

The main function of the outer ear is to collect and funnel sound toward the tympanic membrane (also quite useful for holding up eyeglasses). Whereas the concha has its resonant frequency at about 4500 Hz (just above the top note on the far right of a piano keyboard), the long ear canal has a resonant frequency at about 2700 Hz, about a half octave (four white keys) below the top note on the piano keyboard. If one says the English sound /sh/ as in "should" this is around 2700 Hz (/s/ is even higher at 4000-9000 Hz). Clinically we can place a small probe microphone in the ear canal and measure this. On average this 2700 Hz resonant energy is enhanced by about 17 dB which, among other things, serves to enhance those important higher frequency sibilant consonant sounds. When the entire outer ear is taken into account, the net effect is that it serves to amplify those higher pitched consonant sounds that are so important to the understanding of speech and also for the full enjoyment of many forms of music. In contrast, the outer ear does little to enhance the lower frequency sounds (e.g., vowels) or the sounds above 8000 Hz (where there's less speech and music information). For whatever evolutionary reason, it seems that the structure of the outer ear was designed to enhance speech and music or perhaps speech and music were designed to match the outer ear. Figure 2-1 shows the outer ear, middle and inner ear.

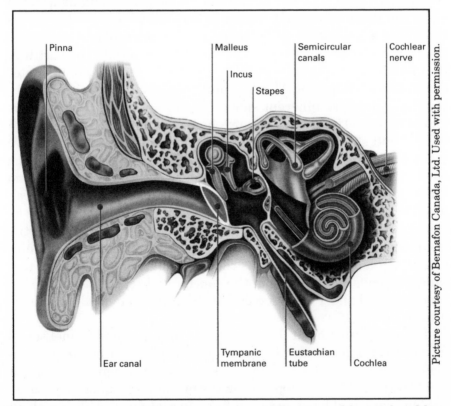

Figure 2-1: Anatomy of the external ear, middle ear, cochlea and cochlear nerve

However, if you're exposed to overly loud music or noise, the outer ear is the first area to receive this energy. Intense noise will enter the ear canal, resonate off the canal walls, and ultimately strike the eardrum. Depending on the level of acoustic assault, it may or may not be painful. The upper limit for discomfort of noise in humans is 120 dB. The threshold for pain is usually around 140 dB. To put this noise in perspective relative to the damage it can cause, we need only recall sailors during WWII igniting the fuses on 5-inch canons, and upon ignition, the explosive force of 190 dB instantaneously ruptured eardrums.

The Middle Ear

Behind the eardrum lays the middle ear space filled with air. Near the bottom of the middle ear cavity is a small opening for a structure known as the *Eustachian tube.* Under normal circumstances this tube is closed, but when you yawn or swallow, the tube temporarily opens allowing air from the outside to enter the normally sealed middle ear. The outer end of the Eustachian tube comes out at the back of the mouth near where the mouth and nose join. On occasion you can hear a pop or crackle as this tube opens, for example, as when flying in an airplane or going up many floors in an elevator. The function of this tube is to allow the air pressure in the immediate external environment to be equal to the air pressure behind the eardrum in the middle ear. When air pressure is the same on both sides of the eardrum, sound can be optimally transmitted to the inner ear. In cases where a person has a cold or an allergy, soft tissue that surrounds the Eustachian tube swells up, such that the tube cannot readily open. The air behind the eardrum is gradually absorbed by the tissue leading to negative pressure in the middle ear that pulls the eardrum inward that can lead to pain or feeling of fullness. In some cases, medical and/or surgical treatment is required by an ear doctor (otologist). This tends to be a problem primarily with children (due to a more horizontal placement of the Eustachian tube), but adults can have chronic middle ear dysfunction as well.

The primary function of the middle ear is to match the characteristics of airborne sound in the outer ear to the acoustic characteristics of the important fluids that fill the inner ear. One can correctly think of the middle ear as a transformer in a train set. The output of the wall socket is around 120 volts whereas the requirements of a train set may only be 12 volts, so a transformation or "stepping down" of the voltage from 120 volts to 12 volts is required and that is precisely what the transformer box on your train set (or cell phone) does. The middle ear is a transformer-like device that accomplishes this with great elegance. To do this, the middle ear has a bridge of three ossicles (small bones joined together by cartilaginous ligaments) which consists of the malleus, the incus, and the stapes (These are sometimes referred to as the *hammer*, the *anvil* and the *stirrup*). This ossicular bridge transfers the sound from the eardrum to the fluid-filled inner ear (Figure 2-1). One long arm of the malleus is attached to the eardrum while the other projects inwardly where a ligament connects the head of the malleus to the body of the incus. In turn, the long arm of the incus is attached to head of the stapes by another ligament. The stapes looks like a stirrup that horseback riders use; hence, its name. The two struts of the stirrup branch from the head of the stapes and attach to the stapes footplate which sits flat on the entrance of the oval window, behind which lies the fluid filled chamber of the inner ear. The oval window is the main opening through which mechanical sound vibrations enter the inner ear. The footplate of the stapes is held within the oval window by a flexible ring of cartilage that allows the footplate to move in and out like a piston; this piston-like movement applies pressure fluctuations to the fluids in the inner ear. At this stage, the mechanical vibrations of the ossicles are converted into vibrations in the fluid within the cochlea.

We have all been swimming in a lake or a pool and while under water have noticed that people talking on land are barely audible and seem to be far away. This is because about 99.9% of all of their sound energy (in the air) is reflected off the surface of the water and only about 0.1% of the sound gets transferred into the water. The 0.1% that gets transmitted into the water corresponds to about a 30 dB loss in sensitivity. For those that like mathematics, the 30 dB loss of sound energy is calculated from solving $10\log10^{-3}$ or $-30\log10$. The minus sign simply means that the sound gets quieter. We can still hear the people talk, but they sound like they're far away. The ossicles of the middle ear resolve much of this loss of energy. And for those who really like mathematics there are two reasons for this. One is because the effective area of the eardrum that vibrates is approximately 17 times larger than the area of the stapes footplate that is connected to the inner ear. The pressure amplification is similar to dancing in high heel shoes—all the pressure collected by the insole of the shoe is transmitted to the small area of the heel (ouch!). In the ear, this translates to about a 25 dB boost in sound energy. This factor of 17 is similar to why a megaphone or cone that people use to speak louder, amplifies the sound of their voice. The mouth has a smaller surface area as compared with the other end of the speaker cone. The second reason has to do with a lever, similar to a bar resting on a fulcrum. The bones of the ossicular chain can be thought of as a lever and the length of the malleus bone is about 1.7 times longer than the incus. This "lever action" translates into another 4-5 dB of amplification. Adding these two mechanisms together results in about 30 decibels (=25 + 5 dB) of amplification and this almost completely offsets the problems of sound transmission in air (outer ear) to sound in fluid (inner ear).

The Cochlea (Inner Ear)

The cochlea is contained in a snail-shaped bony capsule that, despite being about the size of the small fingernail or eraser tip on a pencil, is extremely complex (shown in Figure 2-2).

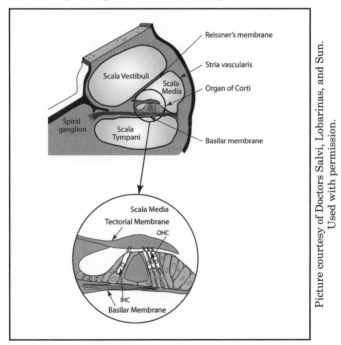

Figure 2-2: Schematic showing radial cross section (looking down the length of the scala media) through a turn of the snail-shaped cochlea revealing both inner hair cells (IHC) and the outer hair cells (OHC)

It contains three, parallel, fluid-filled compartments that spiral around the center axis of the inner ear. The three compartments run the entire length of the cochlea from the basal (base) to apical (apex) end. The stapes footplate in the middle ear inserts into the oval window near the outside edge and basal end of the cochlea. The top fluid-filled compartment is called the *scala vestibuli,* and it lies directly behind the oval window. This is filled with a substance called *perilymph* and has a fluid composition similar to cerebrospinal fluid that surrounds our brain and spinal cord. The chemical composition of perilymph is very high in sodium (~150 mM) and very low in potassium (~3 mM).[2] The symbol "~" simply means "approximately." The "mM" refers to millimolar, a concentration of one one-thousandth of a mole (chemistry unit of a given substance) per liter. In this context of 150 mM, it tells us there's a very high concentration of sodium relative to the 3 mM concentration of potassium. In other words, perilymph, like cerebrospinal fluid, has a high concentration of sodium and a relatively low concentration of potassium. In contrast, the endolymph in the scala media has a very high concentration of potassium which is used to generate the electrochemical potential in hair cells to power neural signaling.

The scala vestibuli, like all three compartments, coils toward the apex of the cochlea where a small opening, the helicotrema, provides an opening into another passageway called the *scala tympani.* The scala tympani, which is also filled with this same fluid, extends from the apex (at the centre of the spiral) back toward the base of the cochlea where it terminates at the round window membrane. The third chamber is sandwiched between the scala vestibuli and the scala tympani. This is the scala media and it is also filled with fluid, but instead of perilymph, it is filled with endolymph. *Endolymph* is an unique fluid with a high concentration of potassium (~160 mM) and a relatively low concentration of sodium (~1.6 mM). This is almost the opposite of the concentrations in the perilymph and as we shall see. This large difference in sodium and potassium ion concentrations helps to "drive" the engine of the inner ear. Along the outer wall of the scala media lays the stria vascularis and spiral ligament. The scala media is separated from scala vestibuli on the top by Reissner's membrane, and is separated from the fluids of the scala tympani on the bottom by a group of cells within the organ of Corti, that sits on top of the basilar membrane. It's not uncommon in the event of a sudden extremely loud explosion for Reissner's membrane and the delicate structures of the organ of Corti to rupture or tear, leading to rapid and permanent sensorineural hearing loss. In such a case, the trauma would lead to deafness in the affected ear(s).

Organ of Corti

The organ of Corti is the transducer of the cochlea. It is the structure that translates mechanical vibrations in the fluid of the inner ear to equivalent electrical impulses that can be carried up to the brain (like an old record player that converts the vibration of the stylus into an electrical signal). Figure 2-2 shows each turn of the cochlea that contains three fluid-filled compartments: scala vestibuli (top) and scala tympani (both filled with perilymph), and scala media (filled with endolymph fluid). The organ of Corti contains sensory hair cells that lay on the basilar membrane and convert sound into neural activity. The organ of Corti extends medially from the center of the spiral toward the stria vascularis and spiral ligament on the outside wall (Figure 2-2). There are two types of the aforementioned sensory hair cells. Both contain tiny microscopic cilia that comprise the transduction channels that allow the outer hair cells (OHC) and inner hair cells (IHC) to convert mechanical energy to neural impulses. The OHCs are located toward the "outer" part of the organ of Corti, nearer the stria vascularis and the IHC, as the name suggests, are located closer to the inner portion (center) of the organ of Corti. There are three rows of OHC and only one row of IHC. The base of each OHC is supported by special (Deiter) cells while the top surface of each OHC is held in place by the reticular lamina that faces the scala media. Further from the center of the inner ear resides the single row of IHC. On the surface of the OHC sits the tectorial membrane. This membrane is actually in contact with the OHC, but not the IHC. This is a cellular, gelatinous-like structure that is connected on the inner side of the organ of Corti only. It is free to move on the outer side and extends to the outermost row of OHC. The relative movement between the sensory cells and the tectorial membrane causes sheering (bending or deflection) of the hair bundles on OHC while fluid turbulence causes movement of bundles on the IHC. Both movements result in hair cell action potentials that send neurological impulses to the brain.

Inner and Outer Hair Cells

Both IHC and OHC are sensory cells with nuclei that are located near the base of the hair cells and with a thickened cuticular plate located at the apical (tip) end. Proteins serve to maintain hair cell rigidity (e.g., actin in the OHC) and both have microscopically small side links that serve to join adjacent hair cells bundles together such that the bundles move as a unit. However, IHC and OHC differ in shape and function. The hair cell bundles in the OHC are in the shape of a "W" while those of the IHC form a gently curving arc (Figure 2-3a). The heights of the hair cell bundles are arranged in a staircase pattern with the tallest row being closest to the stria vascularis and the shortest being closest to the central portion of the cochlea. The OHC are cylindrically shaped while the IHC are pear-shaped. The bundles of hairs (stereocilia) on the surface of both IHC and OHC are shown in Figure 2-3.

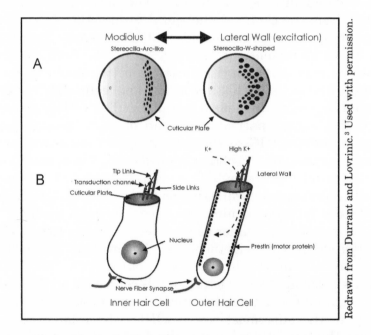

Figure 2-3: (a) apical surface (from the top) of inner hair cell (left) and outer hair cell (right) showing arrangement of stereocilia bundle; (b) radial view (from the side) showing pear-shaped cell body of inner hair cell and the cylindrical shape of outer hair cell[3]

How the Sensory Hair Cells Work

Sensory hair cells also use a microscopically small link (called a *tip link*) attached to a gate that covers a channel opening near the tip of the hair cell bundle. The opposite end to the tip link is connected to an adjacent taller hair cell bundle closer to the stria vascularis (outer portion of the inner ear). When the hair cell bundle is displaced toward the tallest row of stereocilia, tension is applied to the tip link that pulls the gate open allowing potassium ions in the scala media to flow through the channel opening and into the hair cells. When the hair cell bundles are displaced in the opposite direction, tension on the tip link is relieved allowing the channel opening to close and stopping the influx of potassium into the hair cells.[4] When potassium ions are allowed to flow into the hair cell bundle, the hair cell depolarizes. The reason why potassium ions flow into the cell is the same reason that water falls down a cliff—the gradient is from high to low and this is true whether its water, ions, or even an electrical flow. In this case the potassium ions flow into the cell because the relative concentration of potassium is higher in the endolymph outside the cell than inside the cell. In addition, there's an electrical gradient with the voltage being higher (+80 mV) in the endolymph outside of the cell versus (-60 mV) inside the cell. In both cases, the inward flow of potassium ions seek to re-establish concentrations and voltage differences between the endolymph and inside the hair cell. This establishes a receptor potential—the first step in the transduction of neurological energy up to the brain.

Why Do We Have Both OHC and IHC?

Scientists have spent a good portion of their research careers examining the physiology and numbers of these microscopically small hair cells in the cochlea. Estimates vary but each cochlea has approximately 15,000 hair cells (3,000 inner and 12,000 outer). An interesting finding is that only 25% of the cochlear hair cells, the inner hair cells, are connected brain by the auditory nerve fibers which form the VIIIth cranial nerve. The cranial nerves are typically denoted with Roman numerals so the 8th cranial nerve is written as VIII. There are approximately 50,000 auditory nerve fibers and about 90% of the auditory nerve fibers make one-to-one contact with inner hair cells.

How the Cochlea Works

Thankfully, fluids are not compressible (as is air). This allows us to hear different sounds. The movement of the stapes footplate in and out of the opening of the oval window results in fluid vibrations to the inner ear. Because fluids are not compressible, there's no time delay and these pressure fluctuations are sent almost instantaneously from one end of the cochlea to the other. This is why when the oval window moves in and the round window bulges out a bit, in synchrony with the oval window. If it wasn't for the flexible nature of the round window, there would not be any net movement of fluid in the inner ear at all. It turns out that the fluid pressure is equal all along the basilar membrane causing it to move in a traveling wave pattern along its entire length. This was first recorded by von Bekesy, a scientist who won the Nobel Prize in Medicine for this discovery.[5] As the wave travels, there's a pressure peak to this wave that occurs at certain points along the basilar membrane that is related to the frequency of the sound that created it. The peak in the traveling wave first shows up near the basal end (near the oval window and stapes footplate). This is governed by a well-known mechanical principle. The basilar membrane is actually stiffer (less massive) near the base (near the oval window) and less stiff (more massive) nearer the apex. The lower mass near the basal end can respond sooner than the higher mass segment of the basilar membrane found near the apical end. That is, there's more impedance (resisting force) near the base than the apex so the wave travels along an impedance gradient from the high impedance end to low impedance end (like water falls down a cliff, not up). This is like the situation in an ocean where the waves do not continue forever; the thick fluid drag of the perilymph and endolymph serve to dampen out the traveling wave.

To make matters even more exciting, the point where the lowest impedance occurs has the greatest amplitude (height) of the traveling wave. This is shown in figure 2-4 where a certain frequency has a small amplitude (near the oval window), gradually increasing to a maximum (at the point of lowest impedance) and then rapidly falling off. In Figure 2-4 this is shown for frequencies of 8000 Hz, 2000 Hz, and 200 Hz. The amplitude or height of the traveling wave is shown by displacement and measured in what we call nanometers (nm =0.000, 000,001 m)—truly a microscopic scale.

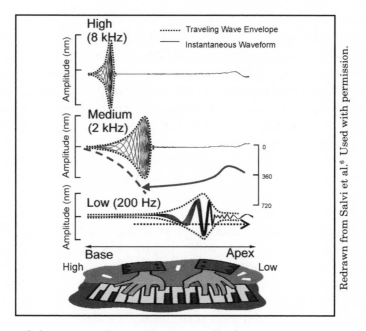

Figure 2-4: Schematics of traveling wave displacement along the basilar membrane (base to apex), for high frequency tones (8000 Hz), mid frequency tones (2000 Hz) and low frequency tones (200 Hz)[6]

The dotted lines show the envelope of the basilar membrane response; note that the peak of the envelope is located near the base of the cochlea for high frequencies and near the apex for low frequencies. The thin lines show the instantaneous waveform of the traveling wave at different times. The piano keyboard below illustrates the tonotopic organization of the cochlea where high frequencies are coded near the base and low frequencies are coded near the apex.

The thin lines show the instantaneous amplitude waveform (snapshots at discrete time points in the stimulus cycle) at several time points while the dotted line shows the basilar membrane displacement envelope over many time points. The peak of the displacement envelope for the 8000 Hz tone is located near the base, the peak for 2000 Hz is located near the middle of the cochlea, and the peak for 200 Hz is located near the apex. The picture of a piano keyboard in Figure 2-4 demonstrates that high frequency sounds have their maximum amplitude displacement near the basal end of the cochlea and low frequency sounds have their maximum amplitude displacement near the apical end. This is sometimes referred to as the *tonotopic* (frequency versus place) *organization of the cochlea.*

Now you should understand that if a painfully loud noise is sent through the hearing pathway into the cochlea, hair cells corresponding to the frequencies of this noise can be weakened, damaged or even dislodged and destroyed. This is irreparable damage resulting in immediate and permanent sensorineural hearing loss.

To summarize, the cochlea acts like a spectrum analyzer that distributes the frequency components in a sound to different regions of the cochlea. The tonotopic organization of the auditory system is established in the cochlea. However, caution must be exercised here since intense low frequency sounds will cause some vibration to occur in the high frequency region (basal end) of the cochlea. That is, all low frequency sounds must first pass by the basal region of the cochlea (albeit at low amplitude) despite this region being responsible for transducing higher frequency sounds. This is one reason why intense, low frequency (e.g., background) noise tends to cover up (or mask) higher frequency consonant sounds (e.g., /c/ or /t/) that are responsible for distinguishing cat from tat. The low frequency masking noise from an air conditioner or a car traveling down a road masks the consonants and this accounts for why many people have difficulty hearing in noisy environments. More on this will be covered in Chapter 5.

Auditory Nerve Fiber Responses

There are a series of cranial nerves that go up to the brain and are responsible for our senses such as vision and hearing. The eighth cranial nerve (again as a reminder, it is written with the Roman numerals VIIIth) is responsible for hearing (and balance). The cell bodies of the auditory part of the VIIIth cranial nerve are arranged in a spiral ganglion that lay medial to the IHC. The spiral ganglion neurons are bipolar, one arm reaches out to contact the IHC and the opposite arm projects medially to form the fiber bundle of the auditory portion of the VIIIth cranial nerve. There are roughly 50,000 nerve fibers in the human auditory nerve.

Since most auditory nerve fibers (~90%) make one-to-one synaptic contact with a single IHC[7], the neural response of each nerve fiber reflects the output from a well-defined region of the cochlea. The lowest intensity of the tone burst needed to activate the fiber at different frequencies is different. These neural properties are referred to as "tuning curves" much like a radio station that is tuned to a certain frequency on the radio dial. A radio station at 105.6 MHz on the FM dial is of course best heard at 105.6 MHz, however, if the volume is high enough (and you live in an area that is not too crowded with radio signals) you may be able to hear the radio station at 105.7 or 105.8 MHz as well. Auditory nerve fibers are tuned very precisely to respond best to a certain frequency (called the *characteristic frequency*—CF), but if the input stimulus is intense enough that nerve fiber will fire off a response towards the brain if the stimulus is a nearby frequency as well. The sound intensity needed to produce a threshold response increases rapidly as the frequency moves above. As the frequency moves below CF, the sound intensity needed to elicit a response initially increases rapidly; however, the increase in threshold becomes more gradual 1-2 octaves below CF resulting in a more broadly tuned, low frequency tail. Thus, the typical auditory nerve fiber has a low threshold, narrowly tuned tip flanked by a steeply rising slope on the high-frequency side of CF. The slope below CF initial rises steeply, but then flattens out to form a high-thresholds broadly tuned tail.

The tuning curve of each auditory nerve fiber is focused on a narrow range of frequencies. However, humans can hear over a wide range of frequencies because some fibers are tuned to low frequencies and others to mid or high frequencies that span the entire range of hearing.

Central Auditory Pathway

From the cochlea, the neurological input travels to the cochlear nucleus (Figure 2-5), and the output of the cochlear nucleus is relayed up to a structure called the *superior olivary complex*. Even though the neurological input may be from only one side (e.g. right ear) the neurological stimuli will travel to both sides of the brainstem. Comparing the relative intensities and time of arrival from the two ears allows us to localize sound. For example, sounds emitted from a loudspeaker located on the right side of the head will arrive at the right ear first and the left ear a fraction of a second later. The delay in the sounds reaching our two ears is especially useful for the localization of lower frequency sounds (below 2000 Hz). In contrast, a different cue is used for the localization of higher frequency sounds. This is simply that higher frequency sounds "see" the head as an acoustic shadow and are less intense by the time they reach the other ear. The combination of a time delay between the two ears (for the lower frequency sounds) and an intensity difference between the two ears (for the higher frequency sounds) allow us to localize with a fair level of accuracy. The superior olivary complex is the first level in the brain where input from our two ears can be coordinated; however, extensive interaural connections exist at all higher levels.

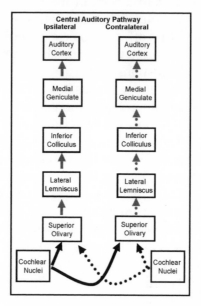

Figure 2-5: Highly simplified block diagram of the central auditory pathway showing the first major interaural connection between the ipsilateral and contralateral (dashed line) auditory pathways occurring at the level of the cochlear nuclei superior olivary complex

Summary

The human ear is an organ made up of four distinct parts: the outer ear, the middle ear, the cochlea or inner ear, and the central auditory pathway that connects the neurological output of the inner ear to the auditory cortex in the brain. The outer and middle ear are merely mechanisms to allow sound to reach the inner ear sensory organ. The inner ear is am amazingly complex structure within the organ of Corti that contains thousands of nerve fibers that not only transmit neurological impulses up to the brain, but also receives feedback from the brain. This feedback loop is necessary to sharpen the "tuning" of the ear to certain sounds, but acts to amplify the quieter sounds that otherwise would not be heard. The feedback does not stop in the inner ear and otoacoustic emissions can be measured in the outer ear canals if sensitive specialized equipment is used. These emissions have taught us a lot about how the normal and pathological ear functions.

Acknowledgments

Supported in part by grants from NIH (R01 DC00630, R01 DC009091 and R01DC009219)

References

1. Shaw EA. (1974) Transformation of sound pressure level from the free field to the eardrum in the horizontal plane. *Journal Acoustical Soc. of Amer.* 56: 1848-61.
2. Bosher SK, Warren, RL. (1968) Observations on the electrochemistry of the cochlear endolymph of the rat: a quantitative study of its electrical potential and ionic composition as determined by means of flame spectrophotometry. Proceedings of the Royal Society of London, Series B, *Biological Sciences* 171: 227-47.
3. Durrant JD and Lovrinic JH. (1995) *Bases of Hearing Science,* Third Ed., Baltimore: Williams and Wilkins, p. 144.
4. Hudspeth AJ. (1992) Hair-bundle mechanics and a model for mechanoelectrical transduction by hair cells. *Soc. Gen. Physiol. Series* 47: 357-70.
5. Bekesy G. (1960) *Experiments in Hearing.* New York: John Wiley & Sons.
6. Salvi et al. (2007) Anatomy and physiology of the peripheral auditory system. In: Roeser, R., Hosford-Dunn, H., Valente, M., (Eds.), *Audiology Diagnosis.* Thieme: New York, pp. 17-36.
7. Spoendlin H. (1972) Innervation densities of the cochlea. *Acta Oto-Laryngol.* 67: 235-248.

CHAPTER THREE

Noise—Harmful Physical and Mental Consequences

Arline L. Bronzaft, Ph.D.

Dr. Bronzaft is Professor Emerita of Lehman College, City University of New York. She serves on the Mayor's Council on the Environment of New York City and was also named to the Council by the three previous mayors. She examines the impacts of noise on mental and physical well-being and is the author of landmark research on the adverse effects of noise on classroom learning. Dr. Bronzaft writes extensively on noise in books, academic journals and in the more popular press; is frequently quoted in the media; and advises anti-noise groups in the United States, Canada, United Kingdom, and others; and in 2007 she assisted in the updating of New York City's Noise Code.

As you've read by now, noise is sometimes viewed as loud sounds that are intrusive and bothersome. You've also read that what may be noise to one person's ears can be music to another's ears. The youngster listening to the popular music of her generation finds that although her music is not being played loudly, her next door neighbor finds it disturbing. Yet, scientists have been able to define noise and when they conducted studies on the impact of noise, they found that noise did not only impair hearing ability nor was it simply annoying, noise was found to adversely affect our physical and mental health. However, before these studies on the hazardous impact of noise found their way into a growing body of research, people knew that unwanted sounds (that's what noise is) interrupted ongoing activities and restful respites and these sounds were indeed harmful to their heads and bodies. Furthermore, these sounds did not have to be loud to be perceived as disruptive.

Yet too often, complaints about noise from upstairs neighbors, outside traffic, overhead jets and passing boom cars are ignored. Landlords tell tenants that they have to learn to live with neighbor noise; airport managers inform communities that they have to adapt to overhead jet sounds; legislators tell their constituents that urban living means dealing with unpleasant surrounding sounds. So, many people begin to believe that nothing can be done to lessen the din. Some people try drowning out nearby sounds by raising their own television sounds louder. Others seek quieter places to live. Still others, perhaps the majority, continue to suffer the onslaught of imposing noise.

While noises intruded upon people's lives dating back to Ancient Rome, as one investigator[1] recounts, it wasn't until the Industrial Revolution and the early 20th century that noise grew in leaps and bounds. This investigator goes on to list the many sources of noise including those associated with transportation, industry, and recreation. She was wise to note that her list would probably be outdated by the time her chapter is published and she was proven right because she didn't discuss cars with their excessively loud stereos (boom cars) as a source of noise that disrupts the peace and quiet on so many streets and in so many neighborhoods.

In the 1970s, the US Government did recognize the deleterious effects of noise and passed the Noise Control Act in 1972. This Act stated that Americans were not to be subjected to noises that jeopardized their health and well-being. In order to enforce this Act, jurisdiction was given to the Office of Noise Abatement and Control (ONAC) that was established within the Environmental Protection Agency (EPA). Although ONAC was charged with setting sound limits for trucks, trains and machinery, it also published excellent brochures and leaflets educating the public about the dangers of noise, and was formulating a policy that would require sound level labels on consumer products. Then, it was essentially "put out of business." In 1978, the passage of the Quiet Communities Act enabled the EPA to provide assistance to cities and states to develop and carry out their own noise control programs. When Ronald Reagan was elected President in 1980, ONAC was "defunded" because Ronald Reagan believed noise was a state issue and Congress agreed with him as did the presidents and congresses that followed Reagan. Although the Occupational Safety and Health Administration (OSHA) continued to monitor noise in the workplace, citizens for the most part did not have a federal anti-noise voice in Washington.

Let's look at some political issues that surround the noise problem. New York City had its own noise code that it passed in 1972, but other cities and states had largely lacked noise laws and ordinances. New York City, even with a noise code that many thought was forward thinking when it was passed over thirty years ago, in response to the increased numbers of noise complaints, reaching as high as 350,000 several years ago, revised its noise code in 2007 to cope with the ever growing noise complaints in this large metropo-

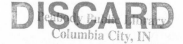

lis. In response to the many citizens who have clamored for quieter environments this past decade and the formation of anti-noise groups,* cities across the country have been passing noise ordinances. However, anti-noise groups are not willing to have noise laws abandoned nationally, especially in the area of transportation, and have asked that Office of Noise Abatement and Control (ONAC) be refunded. Congresswoman Nita Lowey of New York State has been unsuccessful in getting her legislation addressing the refunding of the ONAC passed, but she plans to reintroduce it again and hopes one day she can garner enough votes for the refunding of this office. Until that day, American citizens have to rely on local noise ordinances.

In the meantime, thanks to access provided by the internet, Americans have now been linked to anti-noise citizen groups in other countries (e.g., Canada—NoiseWatch and Right to Quiet Society; United Kingdom—Heathrow Association for Control of Aircraft Noise (HACAN); Tasmania—Noise Tasmania). Being able to share information with each other, including strategies, has strengthened groups in each of the countries. To gain support for their anti-noise legislation, these citizen groups are now aware of the growing literature that has demonstrated the adverse impact of noise on mental and physical health and rely on these studies to support their efforts. Most of these studies have been conducted in Europe (little money has been provided by the US Government). However, with ready access through the internet to studies carried out around the globe, consumer groups come armed with lots of information when they advocate for noise controls. This chapter will focus on research pertaining to the non-auditory effects of noise, with the hope that you will use this information to join citizens already advocating for a quieter and healthier environment for all of us.

Noise and Sound Do Differ

In discussing reactions to noise, annoyance is one that is frequently cited. The individual is annoyed by the passing boom car or the plane above or the neighbor's loud music. However, in discussing annoyance, one notes that to the neighbor the music is not noise nor is it to the driver of the passing boom car. The Federal Aviation Administration (FAA) would say that planes indeed make sounds as they fly over communities but the residents will adapt to these sounds over time and will no longer be annoyed. It should be noted

---

*NoiseOff; Noise Pollution Clearinghouse; New Jersey Citizens for the Abatement of Aircraft Noise; OurAirspace.

that many residents don't adapt to the noise, but rather adapt to "not complaining" because their complaints fail to abate the noise. This too often indicates to the FAA that residents are willing to tolerate the noise.

Sounds and noise do differ in that noise represents sounds that are disturbing, intrusive and bothersome. Sound begins as a movement of air molecules and when the sound waves set up bands of compression and expansion in the surrounding air, these vibrations strike the eardrum which in turn carries the transmission eventually to the inner ear's hair cells. The hair cells of the inner ear respond to the pattern of vibrations and converts them into a code which travels up the VIIIth nerve. The sound is then transmitted to the temporal lobes and then onto the frontal lobes of the brain and is then given meaning—information, pleasure, annoyance. To the boom car listener, the sound is translated as pleasurable, but to the resident who hears it, the sound is interpreted as noise. It is the unwanted, uncontrollable, and unpredictable nature of sound that transforms sound into noise. Furthermore, if the sound comes from a source that the listener views negatively (such as a bar with loud music), then the listener is even more upset. When the person disturbed has registered more than one complaint to the noisemaker, and the noise continues unabated, the noisemaker is disliked and the noise becomes even more bothersome and disturbing.

The Body Reacts Physiologically

Sounds need not be loud to be considered noise. The constant stream of music coming through the walls may not be loud, but they are still unwanted. A dripping faucet isn't loud, but can make it difficult for one to fall asleep. Sometimes it's the nature of the sound that makes it even more disturbing. When Liz McDaniel[2] complains about her next-door neighbor's music lessons, she says: "The scales, choppy and repetitive, have left me begging. If silence is not an option, at least a song with a beginning and an end. Anything but the scales, please...I can barely hear myself think." Ms. McDaniel is trying to write in her apartment, but cannot do so as sounds from next-door intrude on her thinking and writing. Very likely, measured in decibels, the neighbor's musical scales may not be that loud, but they are especially upsetting to Ms. McDaniel.

These unsettling sounds that intrude upon us and which we have labeled noise are not simply annoying, they're also stressful. Day after day, as one is subjected to this disturbing noise, the person's body reacts physiologically. Blood pressure can rise; heart rate can increase; excessive hormones can be released into the bloodstream. The body's reactions are repeated as the noise continues for days, for weeks, for months and longer. When the stress reactions are repeated over time because nothing can be done to abate the noise, the individual can begin to feel helpless. This in turn exacerbates the physiological reactions.

As the Mayor's representative on noise for the Council on the Environment of New York (served four Mayors in non-paid, volunteer position), I'm often called upon by New York residents who have exhausted all remedies to quiet the noises to which they are subjected. By the time they reach me, they are desperate and I can hear this in their voices. More to the point, they tell me of more frequent visits to the doctor, more sleepless nights, and more feelings of hopelessness. Listening to their woes comforts them with respect to feelings of helplessness even before I make any attempt to assist them. I'm not a clinical psychologist, but an environmental psychologist. Still, my interest in the issue makes me a good listener and this is what these people need so much.

The continuous exposure to noise that causes the body to react may lead to a breakdown in one of the physiological systems. Let's look at what can happen.

When Noise Causes Illness

It is the continuous exposure to noise, whether from the planes flying overhead or the horns at the nearby railroad crossing that may eventually break down one of the body's systems that is constantly reacting to the persistent noise. To study the effects of noise on the body, data are usually collected on residents who live near highways, railroads or airports. Then the findings of these studies are generalized to populations who may similarly be exposed to continuous noise from these sources or others (such as motor raceways or noisy neighbors). The strongest evidence for physiological damage are those studies that link noise to cardiovascular and circulatory disorders; some of these studies date back to the 1970s.[3-10] Road traffic and aircraft noise have been found to affect children's cardiovascular systems as well.[6] The US Government in a 1978 document entitled *Noise: A Health Problem*[11] noted that children exposed to aircraft noise in school and at home had higher blood pressures than children in quieter areas. Although the Environmental Protection Agency (EPA) in this booklet cautioned that more studies were needed to confirm this finding, it still concluded that "...this finding is cause for serious concern."

Sometimes, exposure to noise starts early in life; infants in neonatal intensive care units (NICU) are exposed to noise that not only puts them at risk for hearing loss, but it also elicits undesirable physiological responses such as changes in heart rate, oxygen saturation and blood pressure. Goines[12] in writing about the potential physiological changes in infants brought about by the disruptive sounds to which they're exposed informs us that recommendations are now in place to minimize the noise in the NICU units in the hospitals. Additionally, parents are warned not to expose their infants to noise when they're discharged from the hospital. Parents should also be cautioned about keeping homes quieter because two researchers[13] in 1982 found that noisy homes can intrude on children's speech and cognitive development. This points to the value of lowering stereo systems and televisions as well as voices which too often are raised to shouts. The Toronto Health Department (www.city.toronto.on.ca/health) has produced a pamphlet entitled *Noise and Children* directed at parents, and it states that: "A quiet home offers your child a place that fosters learning, promotes health and a chance to enjoy family time."

While one might say that we need additional studies to validate all the findings cited above, it should be noted that William Stewart, the former Surgeon General of the United States in 1978 pointed out that there are many incidents of heart disease occurring daily in the US for which, "The noise of the 20th century living is a major contributory cause."[11] Today, research on the effects of noise on health have been conducted, for the most part in Europe. The US Government moved from a position in 1978, when it believed that there was enough evidence to support cautioning people against the hazardous health impact of noise to the position it now takes which is one that asks for further research linking noise to health. Yet, the US Government is hesitant to support noise/health research.

Diminished Quality of Life

Good health is a state of well-being and not merely the absence of symptoms. Individuals who live with the neighbor's noise or the aircraft traffic may not yet experience high blood pressure or heart disease, but that person is not living what the World Health Organization would deem a decent quality of life. Giving up the use of your backyard on warm summer days because of aircraft noise or having your neighbor's loud music intrude on your conversations or having to miss parts of your favorite television program as the train horns blast indicate a diminished quality of life.

The Okinawa Prefectual Government in 1999 reported that quality of life was diminished for Okinawa residents who lived near the airport because the noise interfered with their daily activities.[14] Similarly, the residents who responded to a questionnaire on the impact of aircraft noise on their behavior complained that aviation noise interfered with enjoyment of outdoors areas, radio and television listening, their right to open windows and home conversations.[15] In a more recent study on the impact of airport-related noise, it was found that while community residents were bothered by airport-related noise and this noise interfered with their life activities, a group not exposed to airport-related noise also complained about other noises in their communities which disrupted their activities (such as talking on the phone and listening to television).[16] Thus, one can conclude that continuous exposure to noise may not necessarily make one ill, but it can most certainly interfere with a person's ability to enjoy good health.

Affects of Noise on Children besides Hearing Impairment

The literature detailing the adverse effects of noise on the hearing of children and teenagers has resulted in warnings that young people should protect their ears when exposed to loud sounds. However, less is said about the non-auditory effects of noise on children beyond potential hearing impairment. President Obama in his speech before Congress in February, 2009, however, hinted about one potential non-auditory effect, namely learning in a classroom, when he told the story of his visit to a school in South Carolina:

> "And I think about Ty'Sheoma Bethea, the young girl from that school I visited in Dillon, South Carolina—a place where the ceilings leak, the paint peels off the walls, and they have to stop teaching six times a day because the train barrels by their classroom."

If teaching had stopped six times a day because of train noise, then learning must have stopped as well.

My interest in the effects of train noise started nearly forty years ago when the then Mayor of New York City, John Lindsay, asked me to serve on a Subway Watchdog Commission. I traveled to and from my home in Brooklyn, New York to my teaching position at Lehman College in the Bronx for about three hours a day on the New York City subway system and depended on mass transit for my other trips as well because we did not have a car in our family. I, most certainly, could provide the Mayor with a passenger's perspective of transit. One thing I observed in my subway travels is that many of trains passed by homes, schools, and workplaces. I wondered how bothersome the noise of these trains was to the people who lived, went to school, or worked near the noisy elevated structures. I decided to focus on the effects of the noise on children in schools and was able to persuade the principal of a school in upper Manhattan, which was approximately 220 feet from an adjacent elevated subway track, to assist me in a study on the effect of train noise on reading ability.

Mean reading scores for children attending classes on the side exposed to the noisy trains which disrupted classes every four and a half minutes were compared to reading scores of children attending classes on the quiet side of the building. Comparisons were done for three years. In the lower grades, the students on the noisy side lagged in reading by about three or four months, but by the sixth grade, the students exposed to passing train noise were about a year behind children attending classes on the quiet side. Students on the noisy side felt it was not easy for their teacher to hear them and complained that the noise made it difficult for them to think. Furthermore, teachers complained of having to stop when the trains passed or to shout very loudly above the din of the trains.[17]

In light of the above findings, the Transit Authority was persuaded to test out rubber resilient pads on the tracks adjacent to the school as a method to abate the noise, and the Board of Education agreed to put acoustical tiles in the ceilings of the affected classes. The result of these two noise abatement techniques lowered the noise level in the classes by 6 to 8 decibels when the trains passed—a significant reduction. A later study[18] found that as a result of the reduction in noise levels, the children on both sides of the building were reading at the same level. In other words, when classrooms are made quieter, children do better.

Train noise is not just disrupting the classrooms in Ty'Sheoma's school, but traffic, train and aircraft noises are disrupting learning in many classes throughout the United States and in Europe as well as noted by the studies following my earlier work. More recently, Stansfeld and his colleagues[19] looked at the impact of aircraft noise on school children in three countries: Spain, the United Kingdom and the Netherlands. They concluded that aircraft noise could impair reading comprehension. The Federal Interagency Committee on Aviation Noise (FICAN) issued a position paper in September 2000 in which it concluded that, after examining twenty studies, the strongest findings indicate that aircraft noise interferes with reading.[20] Looking to see whether children attending schools near Heathrow Airport could adapt to aircraft noise exposure in their classrooms after a follow-up testing one year later, researchers in 2001[21] found that the children did not get used to the noise.

In an earlier review paper on the non-auditory effects of noise on children, investigators[22] discussed studies exploring the impact of noise on schoolroom reading, but also looked at the non-auditory effects of noise on cognitive processes and motivation. These investigators also wrote about the relationship between residing and attending school near a noise source and elevated blood pressure in children, but they determined that stronger data were necessary to support this finding. In a later review article, researchers[6] similarly expressed concern about the finding that excessive road traffic and aircraft noise may adversely affect the cardiovascular system in children. Additionally, investigators[23] in 2009, studying children attending schools exposed to aircraft and road traffic noise, found aircraft noise to be associated with increased scores in hypersensitivity. Another study[24] in 2003, which examined ambient neighborhood noise on primary schoolchildren, found that chronic noise was significantly related to poor intentional and incidental memory. Investigators[25] in 2002 found that ambient neighborhood noise had a small adverse impact on mental health, but led to poorer classroom performance.

Researchers are continuing to investigate the impact of noise on different aspects of children's memory, but the evidence that classroom noise impedes acquisition of reading in the classroom appears especially strong. Undoubtedly, intrusive noise from outside the school building as well as within the building makes it difficult for teachers to teach and children to learn. The American National Standards Institute's (ANSI) recently set public acoustical standards for classrooms in 2002, emphatically underscoring how important a proper acoustical classroom environment is for teaching and learning to take place.[27] The American Speech-Language-Hearing Association's (ASHA) announced in May 2009 that the House Education and Labor Committee passed a bill, the 21st century Green High-Performing School Facilities Act that, "...expanded the classroom noise and acoustics provisions in the legislation." If this bill becomes law, then federal grants to districts would allow "...measures designed to reduce or eliminate human exposure to classroom noise and environmental noise pollution." (US House Committee on Education and Labor). The 1978 Environmental Protection Agency booklet *Noise: A Health Problem* expressed its concern about noise and children when it stated the following: "Noise may hinder the development of language skills in children. Noise disrupts the educational process."[11] Yet, it has taken the US Government over thirty years to consider legislation that would halt the intrusion of noise on the educational process.

The Department of Environmental Protection of New York City (www.nycdep.org) has developed a program that educates children to the dangers of noise and, hopefully, those children in the schools that receive this program pass on the information about dangers of noise to their family members. This program also makes the school more aware of the hazards of noise. The teachers and administrators can be helpful in advocating for quieter classrooms. Cities, just as they have passed legislation to lessen the din, can also engage in programs that educate young children to the dangers of noise. Education is one of the best ways to prevent problems associated with loud sounds, especially hearing loss.

Noise Disrupts Sleep

When the car alarm started, it jolted Alan Feuer and his wife out of sleep.[27] The next dawn, having scarcely slept, Mr. Feuer urged the owner of the car with a handwritten note to fix the alarm. But at 4:15 a.m. the next day, the alarm awakened him and as soon as it stopped, the family fell asleep, but only to be awakened yet again. Mr. Feuer, who considers himself not one to anger quickly, resorted to throwing eggs and yogurt at the offending car and took delight in the way the car looked after he splattered it with eggs and yogurt. Noise disrupting sleep arouses anger and hostility, and can even move good people to do irrational things. Mr. Feuer is not alone in complaining about the impact of noise on his needed sleep.

Sleep is important to health. However, failing to get a good night's sleep can affect us beyond preventing the body's restorative time to heal—it can adversely affect our work performance the next day. A person without adequate sleep may also be less aware of warning signals as they walk or drive through the streets. A 1978 EPA booklet[11] points out that lack of sleep may make people more dependent on sleeping pills. Such dependence is not good for overall general health. "When sleep is disturbed by noise, work efficiency and health may suffer."[11]

Anger, Aggression, Nervousness, Mental Stress and Learned Helplessness

Like Mr. Feuer cited previously, many people react to noise with anger. In 2000, my colleagues and I distributed a questionnaire asking respondents about their reactions to noise and nearly 50% responded that noise makes them angry.[28] Citizens who attend meetings called by the FAA to discuss future routing plans often get angry at the speakers who tend to downplay the noise. The media in both the United States and the United Kingdom report anger leading to acts of aggression between noisemakers and those bothered by the noise. In July 2008, a Cleveland man angered by his noisy neighbor shot and killed several of the people in the home of the noisemaker (www.noboomers.com).

When noise intrudes on activities in the home, whether from an upstairs neighbor or a nearby loud bar, residents get angry and sometimes they lash back at the offending noisemaker. In the 2008 movie *Noise*, the main character disturbed by a noisy car alarm becomes a vigilante going after noisy car alarm owners. Research has confirmed these feelings of anger eliciting aggression. Independently, two groups of researchers[29-30] looking at noise and aggression in the laboratory found that subjects exposed to noise were more likely to administer electrical shocks to other subjects in a group of experiments, although no shocks were actually given. In yet another study, investigators[31] found that subjects shocked in a laboratory and then given uncontrollable noise gave shocks of longer duration to other subjects. They also found that subjects exposed to uncontrollable noise were more physiologically aroused than the control subjects.

Growing numbers of people are doing something to prevent feelings of "learned helplessness," a belief that nothing can be done to remedy the situation, and to lessen the noise from neighbors, boom cars, overhead jets, loud-pipe motorcycles and so forth by forming coalitions to educate larger numbers of people to the dangers of noise, as well as urging legislators to introduce bills to curb the noise. Two organizations (www.ourairspace.org; www.njcaan.org) are battling the Federal Aviation Administration's (FAA) rerouting of airspace over five Mid-Atlantic states that will increase airplane noise over the residents in these five states. They've joined forces with their legislators to bring a lawsuit against the FAA for its Airspace Redesign Project, charging that the FAA failed to factor in environmental influences on communities. Similarly, the battle against the expansion of Heathrow Airport has also resulted in a coalition of activists and British parliamentarians.

When individuals direct their energy toward doing something about reducing noise, their activities should reduce the anger, frustration, and most of all, the stress the noise brings about which in the long-run could be physiologically harmful. There are groups as cited previously that can help people address noise problems. One of the aims of this chapter is to get people to recognize that noise is bothering people worldwide and to educate them that there are avenues and strategies they can pursue to lessen the noise for themselves as well as for others. For example, motorcyclists should know that the EPA has placed noise restrictions on how loud their bikes can be when retrofitting with pipes that exceed legal limits.

Harmful Low-Frequency Noise

In 2004, an entire issue of *Noise & Health* was devoted to low frequency noise, hoping that the articles cited in this issue would bring greater attention to such noise, which often evidences itself in bodily feelings rather than audibly.[32] In this issue, low frequency noises were noted to be associated with vehicles such as airplanes and buses and with stationary sources such as heating or cooling devices. The editorial in this issue noted that some people may be more sensitive to low frequency noise and as a result suffer greater stress and physiological symptoms such as indigestion or heartburn. Some researchers have identified a disease associated with low frequency sounds, namely vibro-acoustic disease (VAD) which could bring about colitis, ulcers or muscular pain. However, VAD has not yet been recognized as a pathological entity, despite the long-term efforts of researchers.[33]

Noise, Crime, Stress and Law Enforcement

Police in cities around the US have noted that some noise makers (including individuals in loud boom cars cruising through neighborhoods), when stopped for noise violations, are individuals engaged in other criminal activities such as carrying drugs or guns in the car. One website (www.NoBoomers.com) reports many such incidents. An article titled, "Noise annoys but it also masks crime and incites violence," (www.noiseoff.org) informs readers that noisy households may be places where children, spouses, or elderly relatives are being abused. The relationship between crime and noise may not be a "traditional" non-auditory effect of noise, but this relationship adversely affects residents and in turn can create stress and feelings of discomfort. Law enforcement agencies should take reports of noise more seriously and view noise abatement as a way of curbing crime as well as making communities less stressful.

Noise in the Workplace

The impact of noise on health has been looked at in various studies conducted on workers in noisy environments. In and of themselves, these studies are important to understanding the health and well-being of workers, but findings here can be generalized to individuals exposed to continuous noise in the home. As early as 1978, the EPA in its brochure[11] wrote about studies that demonstrated that noise may interfere with the work product. However, beyond that the agency noted that noise may make workers extra tired and irritated. It quoted the then former President of the United Auto Workers, Leonard Woodcock, who said, "They [auto workers] find themselves usually fatigued at the end of the day compared to their fellow workers who are not exposed to much noise. They complain of headaches and inability to sleep and they suffer from anxiety....Our members tell us that the continuous exposure to high levels of noise makes them tense, irritable, and upset." Although Mr. Woodcock's statement was not based on carefully collected data, but resulted from discussions with his workers, the EPA gave credence to this statement by publishing it in its brochure.

In 2002, researchers[34] conducted a field study in which they were able to compare two industries that had high noise levels in the pretest conditions but in the post test phase, the researchers were able to compare these two industries after one was relocated to a quieter site. The authors found that the group in the reduced noise situation was less stressed, but the group remaining in the noisy environment did not evidence changes from pretest to post-test conditions. The investigators concluded that environmental conditions do indeed affect workers physical and mental well-being.

However, workers are also exposed to noise in offices, especially open office environments. Two other researchers[35] in a simulated open office experiment found that the simulated open office noise elevated the workers' urinary epinephrine levels and the workers were less likely to make postural adjustments at their computers under noisy conditions. The elevated epinephrine levels indicated increased stress and the failure to adjust posture could lead to musculoskeletal disorders, leading Evans and Johnson[35] to conclude that exposure to lower level open office noise puts workers at risk for potential adverse health consequences.

Workers in noisy environments also are exposed to conditions that may make it more difficult to communicate with each other or to hear backup signals on vehicles or other warning devices. Designers and architects do pay attention to levels of sound that could disrupt communication and have factored this in to their designs. Especially important to employers is the effect of noise on the performance of workers. While exposure to noise has been associated with poor performance in the short-term, it has been found that workers adapt to the noise and their performance picks up, but adaptation tends to have long-term physiological adverse effects.

OSHA oversees safety and health in the workplace, but its major focus with respect to noise has been hearing loss. It believes that engineering controls and hearing conservation programs can indeed reduce noise-induced hearing loss in the workplace (www.osha.gov). However, it fails to recognize that many workplaces have sound levels more than the accepted 90 dB over an eight-hour period (e.g., restaurants, bars) and offers little help, if any, to workers in these establishments. Workers who believe environmental noise has a negative effect on their job performance or their job satisfaction should make their voices heard and communicate with other office workers who probably feel the same way and then as a group approach their employers or their unions. If noise affects productivity and morale, employers are likely to seek ways to design equipment and work space to remedy the situation. As you'll discover in Chapter 11, there are indeed ways to lessen noise.

References

1. Zaner A. (1991) Definition and sources of noise. In: *Noise and Health*, Ed. Fay, T.H. NY: The New York Academy of Medicine.
2. McDaniel L. (May 17, 2009). Her walls were alive with the sound of music. New York: New Times, p. 5.
3. Jarup L, Dudley M, Babisch W, et al. (2008) Hypertension and exposure to noise near airports: the HYENA study. *Environmental Health Perspectives* 116: 329-333.
4. Babisch W. (2006) Transportation noise and cardiovascular risk; updated review and synthesis of epidemiological studies indicate that the evidence has increased. *Noise & Health* 8: 1-29.
5. Ising H and Kruppa B. (2004) Health effects caused by noise: evidence from the literature from the past 25 years. *Noise & Health,* 6: 5-13.
6. Passchier-Vermeer, W and Passchier WF. (2000) Noise exposure and public health. *Environmental Health Perspective* 108: (Suppl. 1), 123-131.
7. Fay TH [Ed] (1991) *Noise & Health.* New York: The New York Academy of Science.
8. Kryter KD (1985) *The Effects of Noise on Man.* Second Edition, Orlando, FL: Academic Press Inc.
9. Tomei F, Tomao E, Papaleo B et al. (1995) Epidemiological and clinical study of subjects occupationally exposed to noise. *International Journal of Angiology* 4: 117-121.
10. Malamed S Fried Y and Froom P. (2001) The interactive effect of chronic exposure to noise and job complexity on changes in blood pressure and job satisfaction: a longitudinal study of industrial employees. *Journal of Occupational and Health Psychology* 6: 182-185.
11. Environmental Protection Agency (1978) *Noise: A Health Problem.* Washington, DC: United States Environmental Protection Agency, Office of Noise Abatement and Control.
12. Goines L. (2008) The importance of quiet in the home: teaching noise awareness to parents before the neonate is discharged from the NICU. *Neonatal Network* 27: 171-176.5, United States.
13. Wachs T and Gruen G. (1982) Early experience and human development. New York: Plenum.
14. Okinawa, Prefectual Government. (March, 1999) A report on the aircraft noise as a public health problem in Okinawa. Japan: Okinawa Prefectural Government: Department of Culture and Environmental Affairs.

15. Bronzaft AL, Ahern HD, McGinn R, et al. (1998) Aircraft noise: a potential health hazard. *Environment and Behavior* 30: 101-113.
16. Cohen BS, Bronzaft AL, Heikkinen M, et al. (2008) Airport-related air pollution and noise. *Journal of Occupational & Environmental Hygiene* 5: 119-129.
17. Bronzaft AL, McCarthy D. (1975) The effect of elevated train noise on reading ability. *Environment and Behavior* 5: 517-528.
18. Bronzaft AL. (1981) The effect of a noise abatement program on reading ability. *Journal of Environmental Psychology* 1: 215-222.
19. Stansfeld SA, Berglund B, Clark C. et al. (2005) Aircraft and road traffic noise and children's cognition and health: a cross-national study. *Lancet* 365:1942-1949.
20. Federal Interagency Committee on Aircraft Noise (FICAN). (2000) FICAN position on research effects of aircraft noise on classroom learning. Washington DC: Federal Interagency Committee on Aviation Noise.
21. Haines MM, Stansfeld SA, Soames Job RF, et al. (2001) A follow-up study of effects of chronic aircraft noise exposure on child stress responses and cognition. *International Journal of Epidemiology* 30: 839-845.
22. Evans GW, Lepore SJ (1993) Non-auditory effects of noise on children; a critical review. *Children's Environments* 10: 42-72.
23. Stansfeld SA, Clark C, Cameron RM, et al. (2009) Aircraft and road traffic noise exposure and children's mental health. *Journal of Environmental Psychology* doi:10.1015/j.envp.2009.
24. Lercher P, Evans GW and Meis M. (2003) Ambient noise and cognitive processes among primary schoolchildren. *Environment and Behavior* 35: 725-735.
25. Lercher P, Evans GW, Meis M, et al. (2002) Ambient neighbourhood noise and children's mental health. *Occupational and Environmental Medicine* 59: 380-386.
26. ANSI (American National Standards Institute). (2002) American National Standard Acoustical Performance Criteria. Design Requirements and Guidelines for Schools. ANSI S12. 60-2002. New York: ANSI.
27. Feuer A. (May 24, 2009) A hot night, a car alarm and a recipe for silence. New York: New York Times, MB10.
28. Bronzaft AL, Deignan E, Bat-Chava Y, et al. (2000) Intrusive community noises yield more complaints. *Hearing Rehabilitation Quarterly* 23: 6-12, 29.
29. Geen RG and O'Neal EC (1969) Activation of cue-elicited ag-

gression on general arousal. *Journal of Personality & Social Psychology* 11:289-292.

30. Geen RG and McCown EJ. (1984) Effects of noise on aggression and physiological arousal. *Motivation and Emotion* 8: 231-241.

31. Donnerstein E and Wilson DW. (1976) Effects of noise and perceived control on ongoing and subsequent aggressive behavior. *Journal of Personality and Social Psychology* 34: 774-781.

32. *Noise & Health.* (2004) April-June: 6, Issue 23.

33. Castelo Branco, NAA and Alves-Pereira A. (2004) Vibroacoustic disease. *Noise & Health* 6: 3-20.

34. Raffaello M and Maass A. (2002) Chronic noise in industry: The effect on satisfaction, stress symptoms and company attachment. *Environment and Behavior* 34: 651-671.

35. Evans GW and Johnson D. (2000) Stress and open-office noise. *Journal of Applied Psychology* 5: 779-783.

Suggested Websites

www.city.toronto.on.ca/health
www.njcaan.org
www.noboomers.com
www.noiseoff.org
www.nonoise.org
www.nycdep.org
www.osha.gov
www.ourairspace.org
www.ukna.org.uk

CHAPTER FOUR

Recreational Noise

Brian J. Fligor, Sc.D.

Dr. Fligor is the director of Diagnostic Audiology at Children's Hospital Boston (CHB) and holds a faculty appointment in the Department of Otology and Laryngology at Harvard Medical School. His research interests include investigating causes of acquired hearing loss, particularly in the pediatric population. His work on potential for noise-induced hearing loss from using personal listening devices with headphones has received considerable popular media attention, including being spoofed on David Letterman's show in 2005. Dr. Fligor began the Musicians' Hearing Program at CHB in 2009, enrolling musicians and music enthusiasts in Hearing Loss Prevention Programs to address the listening needs of this passionate sector while mitigating the risk of hearing loss from music and other recreational sound sources.

Introduction

Industrialized countries have made remarkable economic progress since the middle of the 20th century. Much of the economic success has been fueled by noisy industries, which gave rise to a huge middle class. The result is that we have had decades of a relatively stable workforce with a steady paycheck and disposable income to engage in recreational pursuits outside of work. People employed in manufacturing, construction, transportation, and mining have been able to afford a house, a car, and have a little money left over to have some fun on evenings and weekends. While the paycheck is necessary, many jobs do require workers to be around loud sound for long periods of time. Since the Middle Ages, we've known that blacksmiths were at risk for hearing problems because of hammering away at metal all day. In the 1800s, "boilermaker's deafness" was reported in men working in steam boiler shops, for the same reason (metal hitting against metal, and the resulting constant loud noise). Thankfully, the risk for hearing loss associated with noise in the workplace is fairly well understood now and government regulations are in place to limit the risk prolonged noise poses to the individual worker. While the effectiveness of those work-based hearing loss prevention programs is a matter of continuous scrutiny, a less-often studied issue is what people do when they are not on the job. How do they spend that disposable income? Recreational activities such as hunting (and other recreational shooting), hobby woodworking, snowmobiling and four-wheeling, going to sporting events and NASCAR races, and listening to music (either at a concert or through headphones or in-ear earphones) all contribute to a person's lifetime sound exposure. Oftentimes, we use sound to combat the intrusion of someone else's noise, such as a person living in the city turning the television on at night to block out overnight traffic noise, or a teenager turning up headphones to block out the "Easy Listening" station his parents have on the car stereo. Our world is a noisy place, by our own doing.

Hearing Loss from Sound Exposure

Much of this topic is covered in greater detail in other chapters, but the basics are covered here for the sake of putting recreational noise exposure in perspective. Permanent hearing loss can occur when a person is exposed to sufficiently high levels of noise for a long enough period of time. This fact has been known for a very long time and protections have been put into place for the most commonly noise-exposed population: people in the military and people working in noisy industries. The most widely known federal regulation protecting against occupational noise-induced hearing loss (NIHL) is the Hearing Conservation Act of 1983, and the Occupational Safety and Health Administration (OSHA) is tasked with its enforcement.[1] This piece of legislation sets a maximum allowable noise dose (which describes the combination of sound level and the amount of time a person is exposed) to protect a large percentage of people. However, these regulations set only minimum safety standards, only apply to the occupational setting, and, per OSHA, admittedly do not protect a significant subset of the population. Even with protections in place for the workforce, NIHL is the second most common form of acquired hearing loss, second only to age-related hearing loss. Additionally, the National Institutes of Health (NIH) have acknowledged that non-occupational noise exposure is a significant threat that affects the hearing of children, adolescents, and adults.[2] Other, more conservative standards are used in some countries, and are recommended for non-workers, such as children.

NIHL is a permanent hearing loss caused by damage to the inner ear, and is cumulative throughout one's lifetime. The most common cause is from extended exposures to moderately intense sound levels, above 80-85 dBA (A-weighted decibels sound pressure level), and develops insidiously over months or years. This type of gradually developing NIHL occurs when the sensory cells in the inner ear are overworked and die (see Chapter 2 for greater detail on how this happens). These cells are not replaced by new sensory cells in the inner ear, and so the resulting hearing loss is permanent. For more intense exposures, such as from impulsive noises of 132 dB and higher[3] or very high-level continuous noise,[4] damage occurs not only because of overworked sensory cells, but because the sound pressure passing into the inner ear is sufficient to tear apart the fragile structures that are responsible for hearing. This type of damage is also permanent and can occur immediately after a single exposure to such intense sound levels, and as you may have read in this book already, is referred to as *acoustic trauma.*

For gradually developing NIHL, the amount of hearing loss depends on the intensity of the sound level (measured in units of dBA) and the length of time of the noise exposure. These two factors together make up the "noise dose," which describes the total exposure: the higher the sound level and the longer the duration, the higher the noise dose. The noise dose can be reported as a percentage, where a daily noise dose of 100% is the maximum allowable noise dose a person can be exposed to on a given day. The risk for NIHL is different from one person to the next though, because of a phenomenon known as *individual susceptibility.*[5] Two people can be exposed to the same noise dose and end up with very different degrees of hearing loss, because in the total population, there is a range from "tough ears" to "tender ears." Currently, it's not possible to predict who has tough ears and who has tender ears until after the damage has occurred. Given that there's variability from person to person in the risk of sustaining a hearing loss, there are different scales used to determine what constitutes a maximum noise dose.

Both gradually developing NIHL and acoustic trauma are characterized by temporarily "muffled" hearing and ringing in the ears (known as *tinnitus*) that is at its worst shortly after the event and then improves if the ears have a chance to take a break from loud sound. These temporary symptoms indicate the noise dose was sufficient to damage hearing. The amount of time it takes for hearing to recover (which may take hours, days, or weeks) and the amount of hearing loss that remains (the residual hearing loss that is permanent) depends on the noise dose. Decreased hearing sensitivity and tinnitus are not the only injuries caused by high sound exposure. Hypersensitivity to sound (termed *hyperacusis*) happens in some people with NIHL (with or without an actual shift in their threshold of hearing). This disorder is characterized by sound that is loud, but tolerable to most people with good hearing, and is painfully loud and intolerable to the person with hyperacusis. This is discussed in more detail in chapter 7. Abnormal pitch perception between the two ears can also occur, a disorder known as *diplacusis*. In a person with diplacusis, a sound of a certain pitch in one ear is a little different from the pitch he or she hears in the other ear. This creates a distorted sound perception, and is potentially career-ending for a musician, as it would make tuning an instrument or singing on pitch extremely difficult.

What are the Risks of Recreational Noise Exposure?

Estimates of recreational sound exposure sufficient to pose a risk to hearing are exceedingly difficult to make. In 1981, the U.S. Environmental Protection Agency (EPA) estimated that between 16 and 61 million people in the US were exposed to potentially hazardous recreational noise.[6] To a great extent, the number of people at risk for recreational NIHL can only be inferred from studies on work-related NIHL. The National Institute for Deafness and other Communication Disorders (NIDCD), which is one of the National Institutes of Health, has estimated that 15% of people in the US age 20-69 years have NIHL—this is 26 million people.[7] The ratio between occupational exposure and recreational exposure as the cause of NIHL is uncertain. In 1990, the NIH Consensus Conference on NIHL estimated that ten million of these people are thought to have this disorder due to work-related sound exposure,[2] and the rest are thought to have NIHL due to recreational exposures. In addition, it is estimated that at least 5.2 million children and teenagers (ages 6-19 years) have early NIHL. This is 12.5% of the pre-adult US population[8] and it's highly unlikely that many of them have NIHL due to work exposures. In the US workforce, an estimated 30-50 million people are regularly exposed to sound levels in excess of safe limits.[9-10] Adding the younger and older age groups together, this means 31.2 million have some degree of reduced hearing and at least another 30 million at risk.

A museum exhibit at the Oregon Museum of Science and Industry, named "Dangerous Decibels," is an excellent resource for looking at the scope of the problem of NIHL in younger and older people. A part of the Dangerous Decibels exhibit, called *Listen Up!*, invites visitors to test their hearing and voluntarily answer questions about the types of noises to which they've been exposed. This interactive exhibit is not a complete hearing test; rather it tests for the softest sound a person can hear at a single frequency (4000 Hz) which is known to be one of the frequencies most sensitive to being damaged by high-level sound exposure. The developers of the exhibit created an internet tool where the data of thousands of *Listen Up!* participants can be reviewed (http://www.dangerousdecibels.org/results-hearingloss.cfm). This chapter's author has used this tool and here reports the relative differences in suspected NIHL between men and women and between a younger age group (11-19 years old) who are presumably not exposed to years of occupational noise and an older age group (20-45 years old). Of this older age group, presumably some would be exposed to occupational noise as well as recreational noise, but this group is not old enough for hearing to be significantly affected by age-related changes in hearing. As stated before, NIHL is the second most common cause of hearing loss, with age being the most common; since this group includes only people too young for age-related hearing loss, noise will be the most common reason for decreased hearing. The results of this review of the *Listen Up!* data are strikingly similar to the prevalence of hearing loss reported across the US.

As of August 20, 2009, nearly 55,000 people ages 6-85 years old participated in the *Listen Up!* research exhibit and completed the testing. Seventy-eight percent had hearing at 4000 Hz that was normal, and 22% had hearing that was not in the range of "normal" at this frequency. To be sure that the percentages of participants who have actual hearing loss are not inflated, this author set the limit of hearing threshold to reflect an actual mild hearing loss at 4000 Hz (a threshold of 30 dB or poorer). Of the roughly 16,000 participants in this study in our younger group (ages 11-19 years), 10% of boys and girls had at least a mild hearing loss at 4000 Hz. Boys constituted 6,400 of this group and of them, 9% had at least a 30 dB hearing loss. Girls constituted over 9,700 in this group, and 10% of them had at least a 30 dB hearing loss. The number of participants in the older age group (ages 20-45 years) was over 20,600 as of August 20, 2009. Twelve percent of men and women in this age group had at least a mild hearing loss at 4000 Hz. Unlike the younger age group though, the men had hearing loss much more often than women did: 16% of the 8,700 men in this group had at least mild hearing loss, while 9% of nearly 12,000 women had at least mild hearing loss. The increase in the percentage of men from the younger to older age group might reflect the cumulative nature of NIHL; that all loud sound one experiences in his or her lifetime contributes to how good or bad is one's hearing. These data could also indicate that men engage in noisy activities more frequently than do women, at least in the older group.

Some of the subjects reported whether or not they had participated in certain noisy recreational activities in the past year, and the percentages are presented in Table 4-1. There are obvious dif

During the past year the percentage of participants who:	Young Female	Young Male	Adult Female	Adult Male
Used stereo headphones	83%	78%	56%	59%
Used a gas-powered lawn mower or leaf blower	34%	56%	33%	73%
Rode on a jet ski, snowmobile, or motorcycle	32%	37%	19%	41%
Fired a gun	24%	40%	16%	45%
Rode in a car with a loud stereo	75%	66%	71%	73%
Played in band	22%	32%	7%	13%
Went to a motorcycle or car race	22%	26%	13%	26%
Went to a concert	50%	42%	54%	52%
Went to a tractor pull or monster truck show	15%	24%	10%	16%

Table 4-1: Recreational noise exposures reported by participants in the *Listen Up!* section of the Dangerous Decibels Exhibit at the Oregon Museum of Science and Industry

ferences between the younger and older groups in some categories, and obvious differences between males and females in both age groups. Generally, males were more likely to have engaged in a noisy recreational activity than females. Many more young people used headphones than did people in the older group, while similar percentages in both age groups rode in a car with a loud stereo and went to concerts; there is little difference between males and females for these music exposures. "Young" reflects ages 11-19 years, and "Adult" reflects ages 20-45 years. Males in both age groups were more likely to shoot a firearm than females, and were more likely to use a lawnmower or leaf blower. Adult men were twice as likely to have ridden a jet ski, snowmobile, or motorcycle as adult women, while this gender difference was not so pronounced in the younger age category.

In summary, both young and adult men and women often engage in recreational activities that are noisy, and a rather significant percentage have hearing loss at the frequency most associated with NIHL. Roughly 10% of young people (both boys and girls) who participated in this museum exhibit's research study have at least mild hearing loss, with little difference in the percentage of hearing between the genders. Roughly 12% of adults (up to age 45 years) in this study have at least mild hearing loss, with 9% of women and 16% of men having this hearing loss. Men (especially adults) were more likely than women to engage in noisy activities, particularly shooting firearms. This Dangerous Decibels exhibit sheds considerable light on what we do with our disposable income and recreational time as well as the effect our behavior may have on hearing.

Recreational Noise Sources and Potential Risk to Hearing

As described in the *Listen Up!* research project, many people engage in noisy recreational activities. Most of them do not have hearing loss. There is a world of difference in the wear-and-tear on the ear caused by shooting a single round on a .22 caliber rifle compared to weekly target shooting with a large caliber firearm. The most important aspect of understanding recreational noise sources is that "how long" and "how often" is much easier to measure (and moderate) than "how loud." The intent of identifying the following recreational noise sources is to educate the reader who in turn can make good and informed decisions; the intent is not to suggest the reader stop having fun!

Firearms

There's little question among the scientific community that shooting firearms is the most common cause of recreational NIHL. As noted in the previous section on hearing loss from sound exposures, sound levels exceeding 132 dB can cause an acoustic trauma—immediate loss of hearing after a single exposure. The discharge of a round from most firearms easily exceeds 132 dB, and so it's reasonable to expect that after a person fires a single shot without using any kind of hearing protection, some permanent hearing loss has occurred. The sound levels from firearms are difficult to measure, because the levels are higher than most sound recording equipment can manage. However, those measures that have been reported show some trends. Generally, the larger the bore of the firearm, the more intense is the peak sound level. See Table 4-2 for a general range of the sound levels generated by different firearms. A shortened barrel, a muzzle break, and shooting in an enclosure all increase the sound levels relative to those reported in Table 4-2, since these are levels recorded in an open field. The number of rounds that are fired matters as well, as the greater the number of rounds fired, the greater the risk for NIHL.

Firearm Type	Peak Sound Level (dB SPL)
Small Rifle	140-145
Medium Rifle	157-160
Large Rifle	160-174
Shotgun	152-166
Small Pistol	150-157
Large Pistol	158-174

Provided by Michael Stewart, Ph.D. of Central Michigan University and presented on July 3, 2008 on Audiology Online

Table 4-2: Sound levels for different firearms

As an illustration of how common hearing loss is in people who shoot firearms, consider a study conducted by audiologists at Central Michigan University in the early 2000s.[11] The researchers approached people as they entered a large northern Michigan sporting good store the weekend before deer hunting season, and asked them to participate in the study. A total of 232 people (187 men and 45 women) were included in the study. All had shot firearms in the past year; the average number of shots fired without using earplugs or other hearing protection was 241 rounds per person. The degree of hearing loss varied by age (the older the subject, the worse the hearing) and by gender (men had worse hearing than women), and in all, 177 of the 232 people had hearing loss. Half of the people had been taught to use hearing protection in their hunter safety course, and yet 76% of them had hearing loss.

Woodworking

Power tools are a potential source of noise that, if used often enough, can lead to NIHL. Many woodworking tools do produce high sound levels, while others produce levels that are quite low. Table 4-3 shows a list of common tools used in hobby woodworking shops, and the sound levels at the user's ear. Consider that NIHL risk begins at levels around 80-85 dBA, depending on how long and how often the tool is used. For instance, it would be relatively safe to use the 6" jointer and 10" cabinet table saw for a couple hours per week, while using the circular saw or chainsaw (with levels around 110 dBA) for more than a minute could pose significant risk to hearing.

Woodworking Tools	A-weighted Decibels (dBA) at User's Ear
Minilathe with spindle . . .	60
Drill Press	66
Spindle Sander	70
Brad Nailer	74
1-hp Dust Collector . . .	76
6" Jointer	83
10" Cabinet Table Saw . .	88
5" Random Orbit Sander .	90
2-hp Air Compressor . . .	94
14" Band Saw	95
Biscuit Joiner	98
Router	100
Shop Vacuum	101
Miter Saw	103
Bench Top Planer	105
Circular Saw	109
Chain Saw	111

Levels reported to the author by Bob Hunter of WOOD Magazine for article in July/2008 issue

Table 4-3: Sound levels at the user's ear from woodworking tools

How potentially harmful is hobby woodworking to a person's hearing? As noted, that depends on how often a person does this, and whether or not they use hearing protection (discussed in detail later in this chapter). A study of 3,500 participants in Beaver Dam, Wisconsin, suggested that on average, woodworking poses a greater threat to hearing than most other leisure time activities.[12] The researchers were looking at age-related hearing loss in this population, but also looked at leisure time activities to try to account for NIHL that was unrelated to the participants' occupation. They looked at how many people did woodworking, metalworking, rode recreational vehicles, used power tools in yardwork, used a chain saw, played a musical instrument, used noisy kitchen appliances, and used a vacuum cleaner and hair dryer. Considering how often people reported engaging in each of these activities, and taking into account the people who used firearms, the only leisure activity in the list above that had a clear impact on hearing was woodworking: people who did woodworking were 30% more likely to have hearing loss than those people who did not. While other activities (such as using a chain saw) can damage hearing, in this group of 3,500 people, they did not engage in those other activities often enough or for long enough to predictably have an effect on hearing.

Motor Sports and Sporting Events

Whether riding a motorcycle or an all-terrain vehicle (ATV) or attending a NASCAR event, being around large engines can be exciting, and can take a toll on hearing. Jet skis, motorcycles and snowmobiles all generate sound levels in excess of 100 dBA. The occasional use on the weekends for a total of a few hours per week will likely have limited impact on a person's hearing, but nonetheless, does contribute to the lifetime wear-and-tear on the ear. For those people who ride a four-wheeler daily, for instance, the total sound exposure may be significant. Some reports suggest that levels as high as 110 dBA are not uncommon in recreational vehicles, and in people living in rural areas, it is typical to use them for hours at a time. By some standards, 110 dBA is relatively safe to hearing for only about 90 seconds; this means that spending 3 hours on an ATV on a weekend gives over 15 times the allowable noise dose for that week.

Attending a monster truck rally, truck pull, motocross, or NASCAR event may be a special, once-a-year event. Barring other noisy leisure time activities, very occasional attendance at a very loud sporting event will likely have very little impact on a person's hearing. Awareness should be paid though to prevention and protection, given the significant exposures that are possible; and it's not inconceivable that a permanent hearing loss could occur after a single event. A recent study reported levels at a series of NASCAR events to be high enough to be of concern for people who attend regularly.[13] At 150 feet from the racetrack, levels were on average close to 101 dBA (range 96.5-104 dBA). At 20 feet from the racetrack (the front row of seating), average levels were over 106 dBA (range 99-109 dBA). The races typically lasted 4 hours, which means someone sitting at 150 feet from the racetrack would have over 20 times the allowable noise dose on that day (close to 3 times the allowable noise dose for the week, after that one race). For the person sitting in the front row, the spectator would have 64 times the allowable noise dose on that day (which equates to over 9 times the allowable noise dose for that week). In laboratory studies using sound to experimentally induce acoustic trauma, a noise dose between 25 and 45 times the allowable noise dose consistently resulted in permanent damage to the ear.[4] It is not unreasonable to think that some people with natural susceptibility to NIHL who happen to get really good seats at a NASCAR event might leave with permanent hearing loss if they don't use hearing protection.

Such overexposures are not limited to motorized sports. Reported exposures at professional football games can be 5 times the allowable noise dose, and an attendee at a Colorado Rockies baseball game wearing a pocket noise dosimeter (to record her total noise dose for that game) was nearly 800% (8 times the allowable noise dose).

Noisy Toys

There's understandable concern that children might be inadvertently exposed to damagingly loud sound from their toys, given their inability to anticipate risk. A toy fire truck with a siren and flashing lights might be intended to be used at arm's length, except a child could hold the truck up to his or her ear and engage the alarm, bringing the sound source from roughly 10 inches away to less than an inch away. The American Society for Testing and Materials (ASTM) proposed a standard in 2003 for the maximum sound levels for toys.[11] This standard is considered voluntary, but toy manufacturers are encouraged to follow it. This standard states that the maximum sound level for a toy should be no more than 90 dBA at 25 cm (which is considered at arm's length), and for toys used "close to the ear," the maximum sound level should be no more than 70 dBA. High peak sound levels (impulse or impact sound) should be no more than 120-138 dB peak sound level depending on the type of sound burst. This standard does not apply to toys that require muscular activity or blowing through the toy to create the sound. Parents are advised to think judiciously about how their child will use a toy and consider doing an internet search to see if the toy they are looking to purchase meets the ASTM (2003) sound level standard. One recent study of toys produced since this standard was established showed that of 20 toys evaluated, 13 exceeded the ASTM (2003) standard.[15]

Some noisy toys are more obviously sound generating than others, but the levels produced might be surprising. Toy cap guns and fireworks can produce peak sound levels that are not so far off from firearms. Gupta and Vishwakarma[16] reported peak sound levels from fireworks at a distance of 3 meters was 126-156 dB, and children ages 9 to 15 years old were more likely to have permanent hearing loss from fireworks than adults. Clinically, it is not uncommon for a child or teenager in the US to come to this author's clinic after an accident on our Independence Day (July 4th) where he or she (but, in truth, much more likely "he") lit a handheld firecracker with the intent to throw it, but mistimed the speed of the fuse and the firecracker exploded within arm's length of the child's head. Notwithstanding the burn injuries and the potential permanent damage to the hand, such an accident often leaves the individual with a unilateral (one-sided) or asymmetrical hearing loss (hearing loss in both ears, but worse in the ear closer to the explosion).

Music as a Source of Recreational Noise Exposure

Considerable popular media attention has been given to music as a potential source of hazardous sound exposure, particularly from listening to music on headphones. As with essentially all sound exposures, whether or not hearing is damaged depends on the level and on the duration of use and how often a person listens to headphones or attends a concert. Music is no more, and no less, risky to hearing than are the other sources of high-level sound described previously in this chapter. While less obviously damaging to hearing, the popularity of listening to music with headphones may be a more universal source of high level sound compared to woodworking or shooting firearms. It is the universality of music exposures that has some hearing healthcare providers concerned. By shear number of people using the devices the number of individuals at risk for NIHL is not inconsequential, given that a small but significant percentage uses them inappropriately.

Reports of headphone use vary with age, as illustrated by the data from the *Listen Up!* research exhibit: 78-83% of young people compared to 56-59% of adults used headphones in the past year in that group visiting OMSI (see Table 4-1). A survey of over 1,000 college students at a university in California revealed that over 90% of participants owned a personal listening device (PLD) with headphones.[17] In a 2006 Zogby telephone survey of 1,000 adults and over 300 teenagers, roughly half of adults and nearly all teenagers owned a PLD.[18] Of those who owned a PLD, 52% of adults and 31% of teenagers reported listening for 1-4 hours per day. Media reports indicate that over 100 million Apple iPods® have been sold since the device was first introduced in 2001, and sales of all PLDs are projected to be 275 million by 2011.[19] A study conducted back in the late 1980s very conservatively estimated that only about 1 in 1,500 cassette tape player users were at risk for substantial hearing loss.[20] Their definition of substantial hearing loss was hearing that has decreased enough that it was necessary to use hearing aids. Even with this extremely conservative estimate of hearing loss risk, if 100 million people regularly use PLDs now, that still means 65,000 people would have NIHL sufficient to require being fitted with hearing aids from using headphones alone.

Despite the popular media's attention to "headphones and hearing loss," there are in fact little data to prove that abusive use of PLDs is widespread and will be responsible for an epidemic of NIHL in young people. There is no doubt that PLDs can produce sound levels capable of doing damage to hearing, but whether or not people use PLDs at such high levels for a sufficiently long enough time is a matter of ongoing debate. There have been developed rules-of-thumb to help guide consumers in making better listening-level decisions, and some factors have also been identified that contribute to a person listening too loud.

Since the Sony Walkman® cassette tape player was introduced in the early 1970s, concerns for hearing loss were raised. Maximum output levels were reported to be 110-128 dBA[21] with risk for hearing loss starting at a volume control setting of only 30% (that is, level "3" where "10" is the highest volume control setting). The reports of hearing loss risk continued with compact disc (CD) players. Fligor and Cox[22] reported sound levels exceeding 120 dBA in some CD player-headphone combinations. The highest selling CD player leading up to the publication of the study, the Sony CD Walkman®, produced 87 dBA with the volume control set to half-maximum, and 107 dBA at maximum, using the on-the-ear headphones that were included in the purchase of the device. Using a somewhat conservative guideline for reducing risk for NIHL from using these headphones, the authors suggested limiting listening level to 60% of the maximum volume control if listening for one hour or less per day. This guideline has since been termed the "60-60 rule" to reflect that it was considered relatively safe to use the CD player set to 60% of the maximum for 60 minutes per day. A caveat to this rule of thumb suggested by Fligor and Cox had quite an impact in the popular media: using after-market accessory earbud earphones could result in 7-9 dB increase in sound level, relative to levels from on-the-ear headphones. Therefore, the suggested guideline would need to be modified to either listen lower than 60% or shorter than 60 minutes if the consumer preferred earbuds. The popular media took this higher level from using earbuds to mean that earbuds were in fact more dangerous (they are not, read on), and this study happened to be published just as the Apple iPod® (which includes earbuds as the standard earphone that comes with the device) jumped in popularity and sales at the end of 2004.

As an aside, the Fligor and Cox study was prompted by a clinical encounter in which a 15-year-old boy came to the audiology clinic at an inner city hospital in Boston, complaining of difficulty hearing in the right ear. The cause of this hearing problem was because he had impacted earwax in that right ear. After the wax was removed, we tested his hearing and by accident, found he had a mild hearing loss in the left ear, and the pattern was classic for NIHL. He reported no noise exposure, with the exception of regular use of a CD player at near maximum volume control setting. It seems that the plug of wax in the right ear was actually acting like an earplug, protecting that ear, while the left ear was fully exposed to the high levels of music. When counseled to lower the listening levels, the teenager appropriately responded, "If I can't listen all the way up, how loud can I listen?" This was a reasonable question, and likely not uncommon, but up to that point, there were no answers to be found in the scientific literature. So the work of Fligor and Cox was an attempt to provide an answer, and arrived at the "60-60 rule."

There has since been an update to the "60-60" rule of thumb, because that guideline is specific to CD players. Contrary to popular belief, the newer MP3 players do not produce sound levels higher than CD players and cassette tape players. In fact, the levels are generally lower. A paper published by Keith, Michaud, and Chiu[23] showed that the maximum output levels by current MP3 players is 85-107 dBA, depending on the type of earphone. Preliminary findings from ongoing studies of output levels from MP3 players[24] are in good agreement with those of Keith, Michaud, and Chiu, and suggest that the rule of thumb for present day MP3 players is to limit the volume control to 80% of the maximum and listen no longer than 90 minutes per day, if using the headphones (the earbud) that come with the MP3 player (an "80-90" rule of thumb for MP3 players).

One approach European lawmakers have taken is to impose output level limits on manufacturers. French law mandates a maximum level of "100 dB" from personal stereo systems with headphones and specifies a maximum output voltage to headphones not exceed 150 millivolts.[25] It is unclear whether or not different PLD are manufactured for sale in Europe than the rest of the world that does not have such a legislative mandate. Of additional concern to this author is that this maximum level mandate of "100 dB" is certainly not safe. A PLD meeting the requirements of French law will exceed recommended exposure limits after 15 minutes of use at the maximum "limited" level. Some PLD, such as the iPod,® have a volume control limiter in the software controlling the device, and include a password to lock this maximum limit. A limitation of this software is that no guidance is provided to the user what levels to limit, and considers only level, not duration of use. The "80-90" guideline might address this limitation.

Despite the fact the recommended level-and-time limit appear more lenient for MP3 players than the older technology, the risk for hearing loss may be no less. In fact, the risk may be greater, given the capacity to carry days' worth of music and other audio content and battery life that far exceeds that of CD and cassette players. The greater portability of MP3 players allows the user to routinely use the device daily during activities that do not require their immediate awareness of the sounds in their environment. A very common time for people to use headphones is during commute to and from work or school and while doing office work or homework. In a quiet setting (such as working in a quiet office or while doing homework in a quiet bedroom), the majority of people listen at moderate levels, regardless of the type of earphone they use. This has been confirmed by preliminary findings of Fligor and Ives[26] that have been presented at scientific meetings and is currently in review for publication in a scientific journal. In quiet setting, Fligor and Ives showed that regardless of the type of earphone used (earbud, on-the-ear, or in-the-ear earphones) people set music to the same relatively quiet level. A few people set the music too loud when the background noise levels are quiet, also regardless of the type of headphone. In a noisier environment (such as a typical commute in a car, bus or subway), the majority of people turn up the sound level to be able to hear their music over the background noise. How much higher they turn it depends on the level of background noise. Two earlier studies independently showed that the average chosen listening level above background noise is 13 dB higher than the noise.[27-28] In a quiet bedroom, the background noise may be 50 dBA, and so the average chosen listening level would be roughly 63 dBA. This level is perfectly safe for any duration of time, and is similar to the level of normal conversation. On a noisy bus that is 75-80 dBA, the chosen listening level would be 88-93 dBA (similar to some of the louder power tools in Table 4-3) and is not safe if used for a few hours per day. This is irrespective of whether the person uses an earbud or on-the-ear headphone, because it's the background noise that causes a person to increase the volume control, not the type of earphone. The Fligor and Ives study further indicated that using sound-isolating earphones allows people to moderate the level of their headphones in a noisy environment, compared to their chosen listening levels using earbud and on-the-ear headphones that don't block out background noise. Even in very noisy conditions, such as while flying on a commercial flight, the majority of people who turn their music up too loud using on-the-ear earphones set the music much lower using sound-isolating in-the-canal earphones.

"I know the music is too loud when I can hear their music!" This is an all too common misconception this author has heard from parents, nurses, and even some well meaning audiologists. Conversely, one might ask, "So if you can't hear the music, does that mean it's OK?" Weiner, Kreisman, and Fligor[29] conducted a study to debunk this urban myth. They asked subjects to set the music to the level where they liked it, varying the level of background noise from very quiet to moderately loud background noise, and an observer judged whether or not she could hear the music from the headphones. In quieter environments, the music was detectable whenever the headphone user set the music to 85 dBA or higher (considered "risky"), but it was also detectable most of the time when the music was set less than 85 dBA (considered "not risky"). In louder background noise, music that was set less than 85 dBA was less often detectable, but so was music set to 85 dBA and higher. In the end, this screening measure of hearing loss risk ("If I can hear it that means it's too loud") correctly identified whether or not there was NIHL risk only 9% of the time in quiet, 12% of the time in low-level background noise, 16% of the time in moderate background noise, and 42% of the time in high background noise. Essentially, in all situations, "If I can hear it that means it's too loud" got it wrong most of the time.

Music Concerts and Dance Clubs

As with NASCAR events and other loud entertainment activities, whether or not attending a rock concert or dance club causes hearing loss depends on how often a person engages in that activity. With very few exceptions, a single rock concert or outing to a dance club will not result in permanent hearing loss. Weekly (or even more frequent) attendance could contribute to the wear-and-tear on one's hearing if proper precautions are not taken. There's little doubt that professional musicians are at risk for hearing loss from their work, as they are exposed to high-level crowd noise and the sound reinforcement on stage several times per week. Pete Townshend, from the rock band The Who, famously acknowledged his NIHL and tinnitus in 1989, and helped fund a non-profit organization dedicated to the prevention of hearing loss from music: Hearing Education and Awareness for Rockers (www.hearnet.com).

According to a report in the scientific literature in the early 1990s, the average level of rock concerts was 103.4 dBA.[30] At a typical concert venue (both outdoor and indoor) crowd noise alone tends to be around 100 dBA. In order for musicians to hear themselves on stage, they need to either set the level of the loudspeakers on stage (called "wedge monitors") higher than the crowd noise, or use an in-ear monitoring system that can (if the correct devices are selected) block the crowd noise and allow the monitoring mix to be audible to the musician at a moderate level. The sound engineer who sets the level of the main loudspeakers (called the "house mains") that amplify the music to the audience must set the levels sufficiently higher than the crowd noise. In this author's experience working at rock concerts, the sound engineer typically targets a level of 104 dBA at his or her location. An unprotected exposure at this level exceeds allowable limits within about 6 minutes' time. After a 45 minute set, the audience and the engineer would have a 750% noise dose (7.5 times the allowable exposure). If this is a rare event for the concert attendee, it's unlikely this moderate overexposure will permanently damage hearing. The sound engineer, however, is at risk for NIHL due to this overexposure occurring every day.

It is possible to sustain permanent hearing damage after a single, very high exposure during a rock concert. There are two separate cases this author has reviewed for civil litigation where permanent auditory injuries were claimed to have been suffered because of attendance at a single rock concert. In one case, the plaintiff claimed to suffer loss of hearing and chronic tinnitus after attending a show where he had very good seats at an outdoor amphitheater-style venue. Reconstructing the sound levels based on sound monitoring conducted at the sound engineer's location and his proximity to the house main speakers, this plaintiff was exposed to 105-108 dBA for at least 2 hours, and possibly as long as 3.5 hours. The resultant noise dose would have been 44 to 85 times the allowable exposure, which is sufficient to cause an acoustic trauma.[4] The other case involved an attendee who claimed chronic tinnitus and hyperacusis following attendance at a rock concert in a medium-sized indoor venue where the levels were as high as 107.4 dBA and she was present between one and two hours (for a resulting noise dose of 22 to 44 times the allowable). Both cases settled out of court, with reasonable damages awarded to the plaintiffs. It should be noted that these cases of civil litigation against concert venues involved noise exposures quite similar to sitting in the front row of a NASCAR event, as described earlier in this chapter. Thus, risk for acoustic trauma would be similar.

A longitudinal study of hearing in teenagers 14-17 years old in Argentina identified attendance at dance clubs to be the most significant source of noise exposure in this group (more significant than use of PLDs). Typical sound levels in the dance clubs were 104.3-112.4 dBA, with noise doses routinely exceeding 16 times the allowable.[31] Dance club attendance was in part responsible for slightly poorer hearing in those who frequented this entertainment activity.

Preventive Measures

From these reports, it's reasonable to consider those who regularly attend dance clubs, rock concerts or NASCAR events and the like, should investigate preventive measures to limit the unnecessary wear-and-tear on their hearing. NIHL develops insidiously, so significant hearing loss often exists before it becomes obvious. This type of hearing loss is permanent and cannot be "cured" by medication or surgery. Hearing aids have come a long way since microchips and digital signal processing were first introduced in their circuits, but they don't "fix" the hearing loss. The hearing abilities of a person with NIHL cannot be restored to "normal." Thus, prevention is the key. Hearing loss prevention programs implemented in the workforce can teach us much about protecting our hearing off the job. Occupational hearing loss prevention programs are generally comprised of assessing the risk, identifying technical controls to limit or eliminate the risk, conducting annual evaluation of the workers' hearing, educating workers about NIHL and motivating them to take personal responsibility for hearing loss prevention, and using hearing protection devices when a hearing hazard persists. Very similar steps can be taken in preventing hearing loss from recreational noise.

Parents often ask this author what they can do to protect their child's hearing. The response usually includes they take their child to see an audiologist to have the child's hearing tested, and have their own hearing tested as well. How many readers of this chapter have had their hearing tested in the last year? In the last five years? Parents lead by example, and children are very sensitive to hypocritical behavior. How is a child supposed to listen to parents' urging them to turn their MP3 players down when the parent uses power tools and shoots firearms without hearing protection?

It may be unreasonable to assess the risk for NIHL for many recreational activities, given that hearing loss prevention professionals undergo extensive training to learn how to use sound level meters and dosimeters, and interpret the findings. Consumers can choose to "buy quiet," since many appliances and electronic devices are manufactured with noise control in mind. Purchase toys that meet the ASTM (2003) standard. Use earphones that are designed to block out background noise (this is discussed more extensively in a bit). And see an audiologist for routine hearing evaluations. Hearing screenings in school are helpful at identifying significant hearing loss, but often are inadequate to identify early NIHL. Hearing screenings in primary care offices as well are not intended to detect subtle changes in hearing that may be the harbinger of worse things to come. Most physicians still do not screen for hearing loss. An audiologist is uniquely qualified to obtain a full history pertinent to the individual's hearing health and risk factors and conduct measures to detect early changes to the hearing mechanism.

For the consumer reading this chapter, clearly you are already highly motivated to minimize your risk for NIHL. The key now is to be educated about hearing loss risk and translate this education into behavior that takes responsibility for NIHL prevention. It's not necessary to avoid all forms of recreational noise. Rather, take high-level sound in moderation, give hearing a break between loud exposures, and use hearing protection devices (HPD) when the levels are going to be high for a long duration.

HPDs come in many forms, from foam earplugs to over-the-ear earmuffs to custom molded level-dependent hearing protection. The appropriate style of HPD is best recommended by an audiologist based on the recreational activity and how long and how often you'll be engaged in it. A few general recommendations follow. Avid target shooters should consider using both earplug and earmuffs (double protection). While the sound reduction provided by both is only a few decibels more than that provided by one or the other, maximum sound isolation is necessary due to the number of rounds one may fire. Earmuffs shield a portion of the skull (at the temples) behind and within which sit the cochlear structures at risk. Furthermore, target shooters should strongly consider investing in custom-fitted hearing protection. Custom-fitted hearing protection can be obtained from an audiologist, and involves custom earmold impressions being taken of your ears and sent to a laboratory for fabrication of the device. This ensures a consistently good fit and custom-fitted HPDs are often considerably more comfortable than over-the-counter HPDs. Level-dependent HPDs are a viable alternative to solid earplugs for hunters, as they provide little sound attenuation until the sound level becomes excessively high (that is, the firearm is discharged). Passive level-dependent HPDs do not work perfectly to prevent NIHL, but are much better than shooting unprotected. Hunters who wish to have extremely good auditory awareness, such being able to detect game at a distance, can invest in electronic HPDs. These devices are similar to hearing aids in that they may provide mild amplification for soft sounds (or at least pass through soft and moderate sound without attenuation, as though there were nothing in the ear), and compress or clip the level of high sound. These are a more expensive option, but relative to the cost of a firearm, they are not exorbitant. Compared to the cost of NIHL, they're a trivial expense.

Sometimes foam earplugs or earmuffs provide too much sound isolation, particularly when the recreational activity involves music appreciation. Earplugs and earmuffs attenuate high-pitch sound more than low-pitch sound, so music sounds muffled and distorted. Additionally, earplugs and earmuffs provide more sound isolation than is needed (more is not always better). An excellent alternative is to invest in Musicians Earplugs,™ (also called the ER-series of earplugs) which are custom molded HPDs that attenuate all pitches relatively evenly (see Figure 4-1). The result is music sounds nearly unchanged, just a little softer. Musicians Earplugs™ can even provide varying levels of attenuation: 9 decibels when levels or duration will not be extreme, 15 decibels for most live-music shows, or 25 decibels when the level and/or duration of exposure are extensive. Musicians Earplugs™ should be obtained through an audiologist who assesses your hearing, recommends an appropriate level of attenuation, counsels you on the proper use and care of these devices, and verifies that the devices do, in fact, attenuate the frequencies uniformly. A poorly-fitted Musicians Earplug™ can sound worse than a foam earplug, and result in the consumer rejecting their use. A well-fitted Musicians Earplug™ is an absolute pleasure; live music that is just a little too loud is brought into a loud but comfortable range. An intermediate alternative to foam earplugs for people who are not yet ready for Musicians Earplugs™ are ER-20 high fidelity earplugs. While not as uniform in attenuation as the Musicians Earplugs™ they're considerably better (much less high frequency roll-off) than foam earplugs.

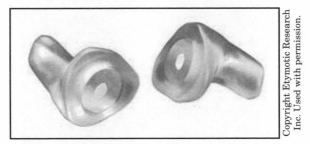

Copyright Etymotic Research Inc. Used with permission.

Figure 4-1: Musicians Earplugs™ showing sleeves that fit in the ear canal and a removable filter to change between different levels of attenuation: 9 dB, 15 dB, or 25 dB

People who invest considerable time and money into their MP3s and downloads should look into upgrading their headphones. Why spend hundreds of dollars on a device and hundreds more on music and then listen with $10 headphones? Research has shown that in moderate to high levels of background noise, people tend to set the music at a level that, for some, can pose a risk for NIHL.[26] Using earphones that act like an earplug to outside sound (that is, block out ambient noise) allows people to keep their listening levels moderately high and still hear everything. There are a few headphone manufacturers who design headphones to block out background noise. Figure 4-2 shows a picture of ER-6i earphones that provide considerable sound isolation to most people (produced by Etymotic Research, Inc.)

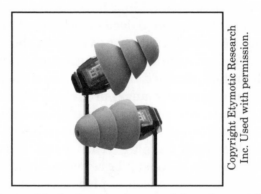

Copyright Etymotic Research Inc. Used with permission.

Figure 4-2: ER-6i sound isolating earphones with universal-fit ear tips and neck cords attached

Custom molded "sleeves" made of silicone material can be fitted over some types of sound isolating earphones (as shown in Figure 4-3).

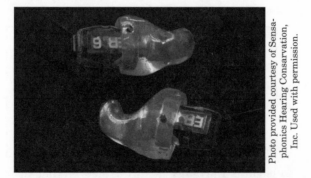

Photo provided courtesy of Sensaphonics Hearing Consarvation, Inc. Used with permission.

Figure 4-3: ER-6 earphones with custom-fitted sleeves made of a silicone material

The benefit to custom sleeves is a consistent, comfortable fit and excellent sound isolation which is quite helpful for those people who have never been able to get standard headphones to fit in their ears. Custom headphone sleeves are obtained by an audiologist, and should be made of a soft material that completely blocks the ear canal. Custom sleeves that have venting (or slide onto earphones with vents in the back of the earphone) allow ambient sound to pass through to the ear and provide essentially no sound isolation. This somewhat defeats the purpose of a custom sleeve: to block out background noise and allow a person to listen at moderate levels, even when the ambient sound is very high. Active noise-canceling (ANC) headphones that employ phase-cancellation technology can provide good control of ambient sound. This phase-cancellation works better on low frequency sound, and requires a power supply (a battery) that could run out during use. By contrast, passive sound-isolating earphones provide sound isolation across frequencies and do not require a battery. Care should be taken when using any sound isolating earphones: a person should not use these devices when there's a need to monitor the auditory environment, such as running through Central Park at night, or crossing a busy city street. Blocking the ear and listening to music will very effectively block out ambient sound, including car horns and ambulance sirens.

Conclusions

Can we legislate common sense? Likely not. Should we try? This might be a matter of debate, but perhaps efforts would be better spent working to educate people so that hearing loss prevention becomes common sense. Legislative efforts to increase funding for NIHL education, particularly for school age children, would be considerably more effective than mandating sound output limits on PLDs. Personal choice is highly valued in many societies, and so personal responsibility ought to receive appropriate attention to allow personal choice to continue without resulting in detrimental effects. Recreational activities are vital to one's happiness and should not be avoided out of fear of NIHL. Moderating high recreational sound exposures, taking responsibility for one's NIHL prevention, and serving as role models to our children would allow us, as a society, to enjoy our leisure time without suffering the ill effects of a completely preventable disorder. It is a noisy world, but we have a choice whether or not we allow it to "prematurely age" our ears.

Resources

www.childrenshospital.org/MusiciansHearingProgram
Simulations of varying degrees of NIHL and tinnitus using samples of music, and the difference between how foam earplugs, poorly fitted Musicians Earplugs, and well fitted musicians earplugs make music sound.

www.dangerousdecibels.org
A public health partnership for the prevention of NIHL. Outreach and educator resources, including classroom materials for teaching hearing-related curricula to kindergarten through 8th grade. The Virtual Exhibit includes some materials from the OMSI museum exhibit, and the *Listen Up!* data can be accessed through http://www.dangerousdecibels.org/exhibitoverview.cfm

http://www.musiciansclinics.com
Accessible information about all aspects of hearing loss prevention which includes articles, FAQs, and fact sheets from the Musicians' Clinics of Canada.

http://www.hearingconservation.org/rs_forKids.html
Resources for NIHL prevention education for children from the National Hearing Conservation Association.

References

1. Occupational Safety and Health Administration. (1983) Occupational noise exposure: Hearing conservation amendment; Final rule. *Federal Register* 48: 9738-9785.
2. National Institutes of Health. (1990) Consensus Conference: Noise and Hearing Loss. *Journal of the American Medical Association* 263: (23), 3185-3190.
3. Price GR. (1981) Implications of a critical level in the ear for assessment of noise hazard at high intensities. *Journal of the Acoustical Society of America* 69(1): 171-177.
4. Fechter LD, Young JS, and Carlisle L. (1988) Potentiation of noise induced threshold shifts and hair cell loss by carbon monoxide. *Hearing Research* 34(1): 39-48.
5. Henderson D, Subramaniam M, and Boettcher FA. (1993) Individual susceptibility to noise-induced hearing loss: An old topic revisited. *Ear and Hearing* 14(3): 152-168.

6. EPA. (1981) Noise in America: the extent of the noise problem. Washington, DC: U.S. Environmental Protection Agency, EPA Report No. 550/9-81-101.

7. NIDCD, Noise-Induced Hearing Loss. http://www.nidcd.nih.gov/health/hearing/noise.asp accessed July 12, 2009.

8. Niskar AS, Kieszak SM, Holmes AE, et al. (2001) Estimated prevalence of noise-induced hearing threshold shifts among children 6 to 19 years of age: the third national health and nutrition examination survey, 1988-1994, United States. *Pediatrics* 108(1): 40-43.

9. NIOSH. (1996) National Occupational Research Agenda. National Institute for Occupational Safety and Health, DHHS (NIOSH) Pub. No. 96-115, Cincinnati, OH.

10. Kopke RD, Jackson RL, Coleman JK, et al. (2007) NAC for noise: from bench top to the clinic. *Hearing Research* 226(1-2): 114-25.

11. Stewart M, Pankiw R, Lehman ME, et al. (2002) Hearing loss and hearing handicap in users of recreational firearms. *Journal of the American Academy of Audiology* 13(3): 160-168.

12. Dalton DS, Cruickshanks KJ, Wiley TL, et al. (2001) Association of leisure-time noise exposure and hearing loss. *Audiology* 40(1): 1-9.

13. Rose AS, Ebert CS, Prazma J, et al. (2008) Noise exposure levels in stock car auto racing. *Ear Nose and Throat Journal* 87(12): 689-92.

14. ASTM. (2003) Proposed toy sound level requirements. Subcommittee F15.22.

15. Bittel SN, Freeman BA, Kemker BE. (2008) Investigation of toy noise exposure in children. *Seminars in Hearing. Noise-Induced Hearing Loss in Children* 29(1): 10-18.

16. Gupta D, Vishwakarma SK. (1989) Toy weapons and firecrackers: a source of hearing loss. *Laryngoscope* 99(3): 330-4.

17. Torre P. (2008) Young adults' use and output level settings of personal music systems. *Ear and Hearing* 29(5): 791-799.

18. Zobgy J. (Zogby International). (2006) Survey of teens and adults about the use of personal electronic devices and head phones. *American Speech-Language-Hearing Association.*

19. Ethier S. (2008) Steady growth expected for portable consumer electronics. Retrieved March 1, 2009, at http://www.instat.com/press.asp?Sku=IN0804077ID&ID=2281

20. Rice CG, Rossi G, Olina M. (1987) Damage risk from personal cassette players. *British Journal of Audiology* 21(4): 279-288.

21. Katz AE, Gertsman HL, Sanderson RG, et al. (1982) Stereo earphones and hearing loss. *New England Journal of Medicine* 307(23): 1460-1461.

22. Fligor BJ, Cox LC. (2004) Output levels of commercially available portable compact disk players and the potential risk to hearing. *Ear and Hearing* 25(6): 513-527.

23. Keith SR, Michaud DS, Chiu V. (2008) Evaluating the maximum playback sound levels from portable digital audio players. *Journal of the Acoustical Society of America* 123(6): 4227-4237.

24. Portnuff CDF, Fligor BJ. (2006, October). Sound output levels of the iPod and other MP3 players: Is there potential risk to hearing? Paper presented at the NIHL in Children Meeting, Cincinnati, OH. Lay-paper retrieved March 1, 2009 at http://www.hearingconservation.org/docs/virtualPressRoom/portnuff.htm

25. Legifrance. (2005) Arréte du 8 novembre 2005 portant application de l'article L. 5232-1 du code de la santé publique relatif aux baladeurs musicaux, *Journal Officiel de la République Française* 301(117): 20115.

26. Fligor BJ, Ives TE. (2006, October 19). Does headphone type affect risk for recreational noise-induced hearing loss? Presented at the NIHL in Children Meeting, Cincinnati, OH. Lay-paper retrieved March 1, 2009 at http://www.hearingconservation.org/docs/virtualPressRoom/FligorIves.pdf

27. Airo E, Pekkarinen, J, Olkinuora P. (1996) Listening to music with headphones: An assessment of noise exposure. *Acustica.* 82(6): 885-894.

28. Williams W. (2005) Noise exposure levels from personal stereo use. *International Journal of Audiology* 44(4): 231-236.

29. Weiner J, Kreisman BM, Fligor BJ. (2009) If I can hear their headphones, it's too loud, right? *Audiology Today* 21(3): 44-51.

30. Clark W. (1992) Hearing: the effects of noise. *Otolaryngology – Head and Neck Surgery* 106(6): 669-676.

31. Serra MR, Biassoni EC, Richter U, et al. (2005) Recreational noise exposure and its effects on the hearing of adolescents. Part I: an interdisciplinary long-term study. *International Journal of Audiology* 44(2): 65-73.

CHAPTER FIVE
Why We Can't Hear in Noise
Margaret Cheesman, Ph.D.

Dr. Cheesman is a Hearing Scientist at the National Centre for Audiology, an Associate Professor in the School of Communication Sciences and Disorders, and Acting Associate Dean (Programs) in the Faculty of Health Sciences at the University of Western Ontario. Her research interests include auditory psychophysics and speech perception, the preservation of hearing function, and auditory aging. She teaches courses in noise-induced hearing loss, auditory aging, and evidence-based practice to audiology graduate students for which she has received recognition for her teaching excellence. Dr. Cheesman, her co-investigators, and her graduate students present their research regularly at national and international conferences. She has published more than 20 articles in scientific journals, served as a consultant to Health Canada and nongovernmental agencies on noise and hearing loss, and coauthored a book on noise control.

We often have difficulty hearing what someone is saying, or hearing someone calling us when we're in a noisy room or operating noisy equipment. If you're a parent of preteen or teenaged children, you may have even noticed that your children, who normally have nothing to say to you, seem to choose the time that you're standing in front of the kitchen sink with the water running, or standing beside an idling car, to let you in on some important aspect of their life. Our auditory system, comprised of our ears and our brain, is an excellent processor of sound, and extremely capable of separating the sounds we want to hear, such as voices and music, from unwanted background sounds. But even this elegant system has some real limits. In this chapter, we'll discuss why we can't hear in noise, what the difference is between loudness and intensity, why two ears are better than one when it comes to listening in noise, and how some useful strategies can help us hear better in noisy environments.

Masking—The Effect of Noise

In order to understand why we have difficulty hearing in noise and how we can improve our hearing in noisy situations, it's helpful to learn a bit about how our auditory system reacts to the presence of noises and other interfering sounds. When one sound obscures our perception of another sound, we call this *auditory masking.* An auditory masker affects our hearing in a similar way that a face mask does our vision; they both hide something from us. The sound that interferes with our perception of another sound is called a *masker* or *masking noise.* A masker may make the desired sound more difficult to hear or it may make the sound completely unable to be heard. Maskers can take all kinds of forms. They can be the less desirable background noises produced in everyday life such as traffic noise, running water, air conditioners or even a sneeze. Maskers may also be sounds that we normally want to hear (music, television, and voices) that are interfering with other sounds that we want to hear. The only thing that maskers have in common is that they're all sounds that impede our ability to hear.

A simple experiment can be used to demonstrate the effect of masking on the perception of sound. In masking terminology, we usually refer to the sound that we want to hear and are trying to hear as the *signal.* Imagine that we play a signal that is so quiet that it can just barely be heard. For this example, let's say our signal is a middle C on a piano. Middle C has a frequency of about 262 Hz. When this signal is just barely audible, we can say that it's just above our threshold for detecting it. Now imagine that we add another low-level sound as a masker, such as the static of a radio that isn't tuned to a radio station. When this radio noise makes us unable to hear the piano note any longer, the radio static has masked the piano note. In our newly acquired terminology, we say the noise has "masked" the signal.

Now, if we leave the static noise unchanged and gradually increase the sound level of the note, at some point, we will again be able to hear the note. The amount that we need to increase the level of the note until it can be heard is the amount of masking that the noise has produced. We can measure the amount of masking in decibels (dB) using a sound level meter; if a signal (the sound) needs to be increased by 8 dB in order to be heard in the presence of a masking noise, then we can say that the noise has produced 8 dB of masking. Clearly, very high intensity noises are capable of producing more masking than lower intensity noises. Other properties of the masker and the signal, including the frequencies they contain, also influence the amount of masking that occurs.

You may have noticed that I have described the masker and

signals' strengths as being their "intensity" or "level" and not their loudness. Sound intensity and sound level are physical measures of the amount of sound vibration. These physical measures can be measured with a sound level meter and a decibel scale. Loudness, on the other hand, is a subjective measure—a perception of how much sound is present. The loudness of a sound and its decibel level often do not correspond closely. We'll return to the concept of loudness later in this chapter. In some cases all that we can say is that as the intensity increases, so does the loudness (our perception of it), but this is not always the case.

Can all noises mask all signals? How effective a masking noise is will depend on the spectra (frequencies) of the two sounds involved and the intensity of the masker. For now let's just consider a rather unrealistic masker that is a noise with frequencies in a very small range—a narrow band of noise—and a signal that has only one frequency. Figure 5-1 provides a schematic of the frequencies of the masker and the signal. The level of the signal is adjusted until it is just audible. The gray area on the graph represents the frequencies and level of the masker noise and the vertical line indicates the frequency and level of the signal tone. We can measure how much the noise masks the signal by first measuring a listener's threshold for the signal alone and then playing the masker and the signal simultaneously and measuring how much the signal must be increased in intensity before it can be heard.

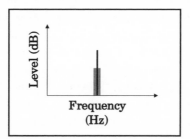

Figure 5-1: Schematic of narrowband noise masker (gray area) and single frequency signal

Maskers are most effective when they have the same frequencies as the signal or when they're very close to the signal in frequency. Figure 5-2 is a schematic to help illustrate this relationship for an example of a low-intensity narrowband of masking noise. The range of frequencies contained in this masker is indicated by the parenthesis symbol in the Figure. If we measure the amount of masking of a signal that has frequencies contained by in the masker (directly below the parenthesis symbol in the Figure), we'll see the greatest amount of masking of that signal. This is illustrated by the peak in the curve in Figure 5-2.

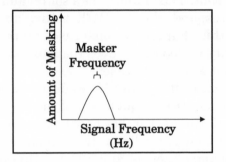

Figure 5-2: Simultaneous masking produced by a low <u>intensity</u> narrowband noise masker is greatest when the signal frequency is similar to the masker frequency

In this example, a signal with the same frequency as the masker must be increased by several decibels to be heard when the masker is present. If we change the frequency of the signal to be slightly higher or lower than the masker, the signal will not need to be increased as much to be heard, as illustrated in Figure 5-2 by the slope of the curve for frequencies above and below the masker frequency. A signal that is remote in frequency from that of the masker will not be influenced by the masker at all, such that a listener can hear it as well in quiet as when the low intensity masker is present. For much higher and lower frequency signals, the signal will not be influenced by the masker at all, such that a listener can hear it as well in quiet as when the low intensity noise is present; the noise is ineffective as a masker. This low intensity narrow band of noise is only effective as a masker for signals that are very similar in frequency to the masker itself.

At this point, a visual analogy to auditory masking may be helpful. Imagine that you're trying to observe objects on the other side of a green, leafy bush. If the bush has only a few thin, lacy leaves, you may be able to see someone standing behind it wearing a bright red sweater. If the color of the red sweater was changed to brown, and then to green, you might find that the sweater became more difficult to detect behind the bush as it became more similar in color to the color of the bush. You may not even be able to detect the person at all if the sweater color was the same green as the bush.

How does this bush analogy relate to auditory masking? If we think of the colors of the sweater and the bush as behaving somewhat similarly to the frequencies of sound, we can draw an (imperfect) analogy. Sounds that have the same frequency are very good at masking each other, similar to the green sweater that cannot be seen well through the green bush. The greater the difference in frequency between a masker and a signal, the less masking will occur, analogous to the green bush and the brown or red sweater. Clearly, the perceptual mechanisms behind visual and auditory masking are not identical; hence our imperfect analogy. However, imagining the scenario of a bush masking objects of different colors is easier for most of us than imagining the masking of sounds that have different frequencies.

The example of auditory masking illustrated in Figure 5-2 applies only to relatively low intensity maskers. Low intensity maskers interfere primarily with the perception of sounds that are similar to the masker in frequency. Higher intensity maskers are also very effective at masking signals with the same frequency as the masker, but they can be very effective maskers of frequencies well above the masker frequency and, to a lesser extent, below the masker frequency. The amount of masking produced by such a high intensity masker is shown in Figure 5-3.

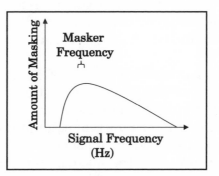

Figure 5-3: Simultaneous masking produced by a high <u>intensity</u> narrow-band noise masker is not confined to signals with similar frequencies as the masker, and spreads to mask higher frequency signals

As a masker's intensity is increased, the range of frequencies over which it can effectively mask a signal increases considerably. This ability of high intensity sounds to mask frequencies above the frequency of the masker is referred to as *upward spread of masking*. If we return to our visual analogy of watching a person behind a green bush, a high intensity masker behaves similarly to a bush that has thicker and heavier leaves. When a bush is thick and dense, any sweater behind it, regardless of its color, might be completely invisible and the person walking behind the bush could become completely hidden or masked by the bush.

The effect that a masker has on the perception of another sound is a result of the way that sounds are processed in the inner ear and the nerve fibers that convey auditory information from the inner ear to the brain. As discussed in Chapter 2, the cochlea processes different frequency sounds along its length, with high frequency sounds activating hair cells that lie near the base of the cochlea and low frequency sounds creating the greatest amount of activation at the tip of the cochlea. When a masker and a signal are composed of similar frequencies, they will both activate the same region and excite the same group of nerve fibers that lead from the cochlea to the brain. When both the signal and the masker activate the same region, the brain may be unable to differentiate the nerve activity (caused by the masker) from that created by the signal. The masker may either decrease the nerve activity caused by the signal or it may flood the nerve response with its own activity. Very high intensity sounds will activate a wider region of the cochlea than low intensity sounds, extending further toward the high frequency region of the cochlea. As a result, very high intensity maskers, regardless of their frequency composition, can influence the perception of a wide range of stimulus frequencies.

We tend to think of masking sounds that occur at the same time as the signal that we're trying to hear. However, the effect of a masking noise can extend beyond the duration of the noise itself, as in the process of masking sounds that occur at the same time as the masker (simultaneous masking). Maskers can also influence sounds that occur before and after the masker (temporal masking). One instance of temporal masking effect occurs when the effect of a masker persists for a brief period of time. The result is that a high intensity sound will mask a sound that follows after it by a fraction of a second. This is called *forward masking*. The effectiveness of a masker doesn't last long after the masking ends, as illustrated in Figure 5-4. The effects of forward maskers are very short-lived and are negligible after 200 milliseconds (1/5 second). It's also possible for a high intensity sound to mask a quieter sound that precedes the masker by a fraction of a second.

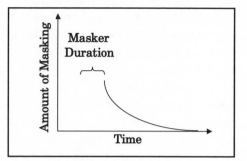

Figure 5-4: Forward masking showing rapid decline in amount of masking produced after masker has been removed

This backward masking effect, illustrated in Figure 5-5 is very brief, typically for no longer than 30 milliseconds and can be reduced in highly practiced listeners.

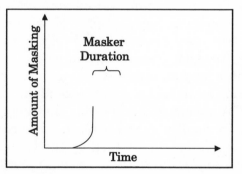

Figure 5-5: Backward masking showing amount of masking produced by a masker that follows a signal

While the effects of temporal masking persist for only a very brief period of time, these effects may be long enough to mask brief, but important sounds such as the consonant sound in a word. In spoken language, people produce between 4 and 6 syllables per second and each syllable may contain several different speech sounds. This means that our ear is capable of hearing speech sounds that come at an approximate rate of 12-18 different sounds per second. When you consider how rapidly speech sounds follow one another in conversational speech, the contribution of temporal masking, in combination with simultaneous masking effects, can be significant.

Loudness and Intensity

Before considering ways to reduce the effects of noise on hearing, it's helpful to understand the concepts of loudness and intensity. The intensity of a sound is a physical measure of the power of a sound. We typically use decibels to measure a sound's intensity as discussed in chapter 1. A decibel scale is a relative scale; it's possible to have negative decibels, for example, relative to pressure like -50 dB SPL, just like it's possible to have a negative temperature such as -15° F. In contrast, the *loudness* of a sound is a perceptual measure that is related to a sound's intensity, frequency, and duration as well as to the sensitivity of an individual's ear. Unlike the case with the decibel, it isn't possible for a sound to have a negative loudness; if you can't hear a sound, it has zero loudness for you, regardless of its intensity or decibel level.

Several examples may help to illustrate these concepts. The first is the case of the loudness of soft music that you're playing while you read. The sound intensity may be 45 dBA, if measured with the A-weighting function on a sound level meter. You may describe the loudness of this music as "very quiet." However, a friend whose hearing isn't as acute as yours may walk into your room and not hear the music at all. For your friend, the loudness of your music is not "very quiet" as it is for you, rather it's inaudible. Your friend has no loudness sensation at all for the music and might say the music has "zero loudness." A second example is one that many of us have experienced quite frequently. When listening to the car stereo while driving on a freeway, we usually turn up the volume control of the stereo. We do this so we can continue to hear the radio more clearly in the presence of the masking noise produced by the road, ventilation fan, car engine, and wind noise. We adjust the radio volume to be at a comfortable loudness level for the driving conditions. Upon leaving the freeway we slow down and may need to stop at a stoplight. At that point, we typically reach to turn down the volume on the car stereo because the music is too loud. The intensity of the stereo that was perceived as too loud in the relatively quiet background of the car idling at a stoplight was, just moments earlier, comfortably loud when driving at high speed on the freeway. Until the volume control was adjusted, the intensity of the stereo had not changed. The same intensity that was perceived as too loud in one condition was perceived as comfortably loud in another.

When judging whether a noise has the potential to damage your hearing, the <u>intensity</u> of sound is important and not its <u>loudness</u>. Sound that is comfortably loud, such as your favorite band playing at a concert, may be intense enough to place your hearing health at risk. Because the loudness of a sound is affected by both an individual's hearing sensitivity and the sound environment (such as the presence of other background noise), we're not very good at using the perceptual measure of loudness as our gauge to judge a sound's intensity and it's risk to our hearing health.

Two Ears are Better than One

Up to this point, we've been considering our ability to hear in noise as if we have only one ear working on this task. However, in most listening conditions, we listen with both ears, binaurally, and our two ears work well together to improve our ability to hear, particularly in noise. Our brain automatically combines and compares the input from both ears which allows us to locate where sounds originate in our environment ("Is the car coming from the left or the right?") and to help us hear better in noise. One of the ways in which two ears work better than one alone is in the simple detection of sounds. When both ears are presented a sound, as in the real world environment where both ears are listening, our hearing acuity is better; lower sound levels are needed for a listener to just detect the presence of a sound than when only one ear is presented the sound. It's rare that we actually listen with only one ear. It typically occurs when we're listening through some sort of listening device, such as during a hearing test where sounds may be presented to the right or left side of headphones alone, or when talking on the telephone and listening with only one ear.

When both ears are presented with the same sound, detection of the sound is not only better, but sounds are also heard as louder. This phenomenon, termed *binaural summation,* in which sounds are louder when heard with both ears, is another instance where the decibel level of a sound and its loudness are different. As a demonstration that you can try for yourself, you can set the music from an MP3 player or another sound system to a fixed volume level and listen to it with just one earpiece. This can be one side of a headphone or one earbud. When you add the second earpiece, so that you're listening binaurally, the music will sound louder, even though you haven't adjusted the volume control. (It's best to do this in a quiet room, so the background noise isn't influencing your perception of the loudness of the music. It's also a fairer demonstration if you can use monaural headphones.)

By comparing the information heard with two ears, the brain can determined where a sound is coming from. We can localize sound because sounds coming from different directions reach the two ears at slightly different times and at slightly different intensities (an exception can occur when sounds come from exactly in front or behind). The auditory system (your ears and brain) is sensitive to very small differences in the timing and intensity of sounds reaching your ears and can use these differences between ears, interaural (between the ears) time and intensity cues, to locate sounds in the horizontal plane. In the situation depicted in Figure 5-6, we can see how the talker's voice will reach the listener's left ear first because that ear is nearer to the talker.

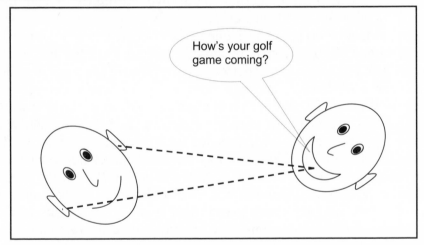

Figure 5-6. Binaural hearing when the talker's voice arrives to the closer ear slightly sooner and at a slightly greater intensity than to the farther ear

These interaural time and intensity differences allow the listener to locate the talker. The sound reaching the listener's left ear will also be slightly louder in intensity. A listener, even with eyes closed, would be very good at determining where the talker was located by using these extremely small time and intensity cues. Interestingly, whether a sound comes from directly behind or directly in front of the listener, the sound reaches both ears respectively at precisely the same intensity and time. For this reason, sounds coming from directly behind a person may be mistakenly identified as coming from directly in front.

Listeners can make use of their ability to locate sounds in space using time and intensity information to separate speech from a noise in the listening environment. In Figure 5-7, the noises are coming from the right side of the listener and the speech is coming from the left. When signals and noises come from different locations, the amount of masking produced by the noise can be reduced significantly, in some extreme cases by as much as 10 dB.

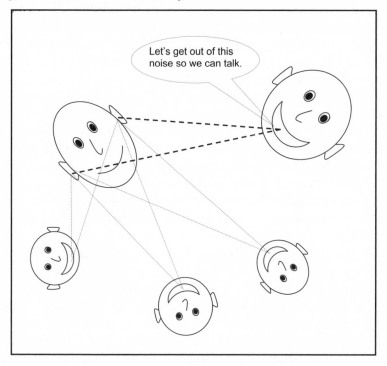

Figure 5-7. Binaural hearing allows the interaural time and intensity differences to separate the talker's voice from a background of noises originating elsewhere

Speech Perception in Noise

Most of the masking examples used in this chapter so far have involved a relatively simple sound, one with a narrow range of frequencies, acting as a masker of another simple sound. However, noises that we encounter in the real world that interfere with our ability to hear are usually far more complex, and the sounds that we're trying to hear (the signals) are rarely simple tones. Often, we're trying to hear speech or music in a background of a complex combination of sounds originating from many different sources. The interfering noises that mask our hearing in everyday life may cover a wide range of frequencies. For example, a complex masking noise may be the sound of the engine of your car combined with the noise of your tires as they contact the road, the radio playing country and western music, and the wind noise as you travel 60 mph on the freeway. The noises may be very <u>dissimilar</u> to the speech that you are trying to hear, as in the case of tap water running into a stainless steel sink while you are trying to carry on a conversation with a visitor. The noises may also be <u>very similar,</u> when you pull up to a stoplight with the window open and the driver next to you is tuned in to a different radio station than you.

Masking noises may be very predictable and steady, such as the continuous noise produced by a room fan. Or they may fluctuate in intensity, like the traffic noise in a busy city that ebbs and flows with the phases of the traffic lights. When in a noise that fluctuates, a listener may be able to make use of some of the lulls or breaks in the masker noise to catch a part of the signal that is not audible when the masker intensity is at its peak. In all of these cases, and despite the relative complexity of the signal and the masker, the same principles of simultaneous and temporal masking apply.

Frequently, masking noises are very similar to the signal that you want to hear, such as the sound of your conversational partner when talking at a reception or in a busy and crowded restaurant. The background noise that serves as a masker may be a combination of dozens of other voices. In such cases, the task of the listener is more than just hearing the speech, it's also extracting the speech of one person's voice from among that of many other talkers. Healthy human ears (and brains) are very good at doing this, even when the conversational partner's voice is well below the intensity of the background noise. The cocktail party phenomenon refers to our excellent ability to hear one person's voice among many other voices in close proximity. To do this, our auditory systems make use of binaural hearing, visual information, and characteristics of the talker's voice to allow us to effectively hear the voice of one talker despite the surrounding noise produced by the other partiers.

Rather than talking about the amount of masking that a noise effects on a signal, it's often more practical to consider the relative amount of noise and signal that is needed in order to hear the signal. The signal-to-noise ratio (abbreviated as SNR or, less frequently, as S/N) is the ratio of the signal, which is often speech, to the background noise. Because decibels are a logarithmic scale (recall your high school math lessons on division of logarithms), a ratio of a 70 dBA speech signal to a 60 dBA noise has a SNR of 70-60, or 10 dB. The logarithm of one value (the signal) divided by another value (the noise) is actually the same as the difference between the two decibel values. Therefore, the SNR can also be thought of as a measure of how many decibels the signal is more (or less) than the noise. A person with normal hearing may be able to understand conversational speech at a SNR of -6 dB or even lower. At a SNR of -6 dB, the speech is 6 dB less intense than the noise. A person with a moderate sensory hearing loss may need a SNR of +8 dB to be able to understand the same speech.

Of course, the use of the SNR to determine how well a person may be able to hear in a given situation oversimplifies the hearing process considerably. As well as the SNR, other characteristics of the signal, the noise, and the listener can influence our ability to hear the signal. Spatial separation of the speech from the noise, the temporal pattern of the speech and noise, the context of the speech, the frequencies of the sounds and the listener's own hearing abilities are all important contributors to whether the speech is heard well. In the next section, strategies for maximizing speech communication in noise will serve to review these characteristics.

Improving Communication in Noise

There are many ways to improve communication in a noisy environment. Some of these are quite obvious. However, no matter how obvious they may seem as you read about them, when you examine your own behavior in a real life situation, it's likely that you don't use them all. (Do you really push the mute button on the remote control every time you're talking to someone in the room?) Some people struggle with conversations in noisy environments and have to repeat themselves many times, resulting in the potential for miscommunication and/or frustration, rather than adopt some of these solutions.

The first four of the nine strategies are aimed at increasing the SNR, either by increasing the intensity of the speech that reaches your ear or by decreasing the noise that reaches you.

1. Turn off the noise. As obvious as this strategy seems to be, many people continue to struggle to understand speech in a noisy environment rather than turn off or mute the television while talking on the phone, or shutting off the lawnmower while talking to a neighbor. By shutting off the leaf blower, lawnmower, snow blower, or radio, you have not only removed the source of the problem, but have also given your ears a chance to recover from the noise exposure.

2. Turn down the volume. If the source of the noise cannot be eliminated entirely, perhaps for safety or other reasons, then turning down the volume may be a suitable option.

3. Move away from the noise. If you cannot turn off the noise or turn it down safely or sufficiently, then move as far as possible away from it. In an open air setting, sound levels decrease by 6 dB for every doubling of distance. So, if you're standing about 20 feet from a noisy bus and the sound level is about 75 dBA, by doubling the distance between you and the bus (move 40 feet away from the bus), the bus noise reaching you would decrease to 69 dBA. This 6 dB per-doubling-of-distance effect (which goes by the name of the "inverse square law" in acoustics), doesn't work in enclosed spaces where sound reflects off walls rather than spreading out in all directions as it does outdoors. If you're indoors, leaving the noisy room for a quieter venue and shutting the door behind you may be the best solution.

4. Move closer to the talker. This may work if the talker doesn't decrease his or her vocal intensity to compensate for you moving in closer. By moving closer to the talker, you may not only increase the level of the talker's voice reaching your ear (increasing the S in the SNR), you may also be moving away from the noise and decreasing the noise level around you (decreasing the N).

5. Change your position relative to the noise and the talker. The situation shown in Figure 5-6 is an example of using spatial separation of a noise and the talker to help improve communication in noise. When the talker and the noise are coming from the same direction, you cannot use these spatial cues as effectively as when they come from different directions.

6. Place the talker in the noisier position (the Lombard effect). A talker's vocal level increases in intensity when speaking in a background of noise. This means that people naturally talk louder in a noisy environment. This Lombard effect helps maintain a good SNR when talking in noise. However, a talker doesn't increase his or her vocal level at the same rate as the background noise increases, so in very high intensity noises, the Lombard effect is not large enough to maintain effective speech communication.

7. In very high noise, wear hearing protection. In very high intensity noises, those over 85 dBA, the use of earplugs or earmuffs can improve speech intelligibility. Why? A normal, healthy ear will distort very high intensity sounds so they become more difficult to understand. When earplugs or earmuffs are worn, the level of the sound (both the level of the noise and the speech) reaching the cochlea is decreased. At very high sound levels, the hearing protection provided by the plugs or muffs helps speech understanding by preventing the ears from distorting the sound. How can you tell if the noise is over 85 dBA? A rough guide comes from our own limitations on how loud we can talk. For example, 80 dB is approximately equal to shouting. So, if you're standing about 3 feet away from a talker in a noisy room and you cannot understand what is said, then the noise is likely 85 dBA or greater.

For persons with normal hearing, wearing hearing protection devices (earplugs or earmuffs) can actually improve one's ability to understand speech. This makes sense when you understand that very loud noise causes the ears to overload, so speech and other sound becomes distorted. This is not true for persons who have a sensorineural hearing loss. For such people, hearing protection devices can make communication in noise more difficult. The need to protect their hearing from further damage, in this case by excessive noise, remains an important but tricky situation.

8. Change the message. How well we can understand what is being said depends a lot on how much of the speech we can hear. It also depends on the complexity, predictability of the message, and its context. For example, if you asked a friend how the commute into the city was this morning and your friend responded, "No good. I was driving in and I ran out of gas on the interstate," you wouldn't even need to hear the word "gas" if you heard the rest of the response. You would still have a really good idea what the complete message was. In contrast, if the response was "No good. Not enough gas," you aren't likely to understand what the problem was unless you heard the word "gas." In the first example, the context provided by your friend was the information about driving and running out of something. This context made the missing word highly predictable. In the latter example, the word "gas" would need to be heard to make any sense of the statement because so little contextual information was given to allow you to predict what your friend didn't have enough of.

The "unh" response of a teenager to your afternoon query of "Did you eat lunch today?" may leave you wondering whether the response meant yes or no if you can't hear the muttered word well in the background sound of the teen's computer game. One word or telegraphic responses that are easily misheard or confused with another word in quiet can be particularly difficult in noise. One strategy that has been successfully adopted to help improve message reception accuracy in noise is to increase the amount of information in a message. Because letters like /b/, /p/, and /d/ rhyme and can be easily confused, the international radiotelephony spelling alphabet was invented. This spelling alphabet uses words such as Alpha, Bravo, and Charlie as replacements for letter identifiers and spelling. The substitution of the word Bravo for /b/, Papa for /p/, and Delta for /d/ significantly reduces the likelihood that these three letters are misunderstood. The spelling alphabet words are more easily heard because they have two syllables and do not sound similar to any of the other words of the spelling alphabet words.

9. Use visual cues. Visual information can supplement the auditory information in a noisy environment.   If you can't hear the difference between "few" and "pew" because of the background noise, a quick look at the speaker's mouth will help. The upper teeth are moved over the lower lip and the lips don't meet, when the word "few" is spoken. On the other hand, when the word "pew" is spoken, the two lips come together to close the mouth. These visual distinctions between speech sounds can be a useful supplement to auditory speech information. By using visual cues you can increase your speech intelligibility about 30%. On the other hand, not all speech sounds are clearly visible, particularly those that are made near the back of the mouth. Visual cues are unlikely to help distinguish "ache" from "ate," for example.

Most people are naturally quite good at using visual information to help them understand better in noise, although some are definitely better than others. In order to make the most of visual cues, of course you need to be able to see a person's face clearly. Moustaches, eating or smoking while talking, and hands positioned around the face certainly can interfere with visual cues. It helps if light is shining onto the talker's face rather than coming from behind; this avoids having the talker appear in silhouette and the mouth becoming hidden in the shadows. Exaggerated lip movements won't help. By facing the talker so that your lips are viewed from straight ahead, or no more than a 45° angle, the visual information will be more useable.

One thing that definitely won't help you hear in noise is chewing while trying to listen. Your ears have protective reflexes that reduce your ability to hear well when you're in the presence of high intensity sound. These acoustic reflexes cause a muscle in your middle ear to contract. The contraction stiffens your middle ear system and reduces the intensity of sound transmitted to your inner ear by about 20 dB. This reflex is thought to be helpful in protecting your inner ear from high intensity sounds. The effect of this reflex, and the masking sound that you create is that you may need to turn up the volume on your television while eating.

While we can't do much about aging, or repair a sensorineural hearing loss if one is present, both can contribute to additional challenges when listening in noise. The extraction of speech information from a background of noise becomes more difficult with aging, in part because many older people tend to have some degree of sensorineural hearing loss. Older listeners may also be less able to make use of quiet periods in noise (the dips in the intensity of a masker). Some older people may also have temporal processing difficulties because of changes to their auditory processing systems. As a result, a background noise that may barely be noticeable and have little effect for a young listener with good hearing acuity may cause moderate or more severe hearing challenges for persons with hearing loss and auditory processing difficulties. An awareness of these challenges and the solutions provided here to help improve communication in noise will help improve communication for all listeners.

CHAPTER SIX
Interaction between Noise and Chemicals Found in the Workplace
Thais C. Morata, Ph.D.

Dr. Morata is an audiologist who has been working in the area of hearing loss prevention since 1987. She earned degrees in Speech Pathology and Audiology, and Communication Disorders from the Pontifical Catholic University of São Paulo and the University of Cincinnati. She is a Research Audiologist at the National Institute for Occupational Safety and Health (NIOSH, Cincinnati, OH) in the Division of Applied Research and Technology, Hearing Loss Prevention Team in Cincinnati, Ohio. Her pioneering work in the area of noise interactions in the workplace has influenced not only NIOSH priorities and policy, but has affected national and international occupational safety and health policies. In 2008, Dr. Morata received the Outstanding Hearing Conservationist Award from the National Hearing Conservation Association for her contributions to hearing loss prevention and evaluation of the effects of occupational exposure to ototoxic chemicals.

As discussed in earlier chapters, several factors have been studied to try to understand why the prevalence and degree of noise-induced hearing loss can vary so much within a group and among groups. Some of the factors studied include variations in exposure, age, gender, race, and general health indicators, such as blood pressure and use of certain medications. The focus of the present chapter will be on the ototoxicity (the toxic effects on hearing), industrial chemicals, and their interaction with noise.

Hearing loss apart from noise can occur after ingestion of certain drugs due to their effects on the auditory system or brain. The ototoxicity of therapeutic drugs has been recognized since the 19th century. The first reports associated the intake of certain drugs such as quinine and acetylsalicylic acid (ASA) with temporary hearing loss as well as dizziness and tinnitus. In the 1940s, permanent damage to the cochlea (sensory end organ for hearing) was reported in several patients treated with the newly discovered drug for treatment of tuberculosis, the aminoglycoside antibiotic streptomycin. Today there are many well-known ototoxic drugs used in clinical situations. Most of them (antibiotics, chemotherapeutics, diuretics and anti-malaria drugs) are used despite these negative side effects in order to treat other serious, sometimes life-threatening conditions.

By comparison, only recently the ototoxicity of chemicals found in the environment from contaminants in air, food or water, and in the workplace, became a concern for audiologists and other healthcare professionals. Initially, there were just isolated reports following acute intoxications, poisonings, and observations that hearing losses were more common and sometimes more severe in work settings where chemical exposures occurred. Other studies on the neurotoxicity of chemicals indicated that chemicals were also damaging more central portions of the auditory system. Following these reports, other research laboratories started investigating the ototoxic properties of chemical agents and identified ototoxic properties in a few classes of industrial chemicals: metals, solvents, asphyxiants, pesticides, and polychlorinated biphenyls (PCBs).

Studies conducted with experimental animals have shown that some toxicants can reach the inner ear through the blood stream. They were found in inner ear fluids (endolymph and perilymph, discussed in more detail in Chapter 2) and have caused damage to some of the inner ear structures and have impaired functions. Some of these chemicals are also damaging to the nerves. The onset, site, mechanism and extent of ototoxic damage of these toxicants vary according to risk factors that include: type of chemical, interactions, exposure level and duration of administration, as is the case with ototoxic therapeutic drugs such as cisplatin (used in chemotherapy) and aminoglycoside antibiotics.

The hearing loss caused by chemicals can be very similar to a hearing loss caused by excessive noise. Since noise exposure is so common in modern societies, this might explain the delay in recognizing the risk to hearing that these chemicals can pose. Also, in most cases, the hearing loss as detected by a pure tone audiometric test is often just mild to moderate. Moreover, the results of the audiometric test for a noise-induced hearing loss and an ototoxic hearing loss can have the same configuration on the audiogram. It is also known that generally, in these disorders, hearing loss is bilateral, with symmetrical patterns on the audiogram for both ears, and is often irreversible. Hearing loss starts in the high frequencies (higher pitches, 3000-6000 Hz), and progresses at a rate determined by exposure to various risk factors. Hearing loss caused by ototoxicity is usually cochlear (that is, sensorineural).

Pure tone audiometry is a basic clinical test that is used to determine a person's hearing sensitivity at specific frequencies, i.e., the softest sound that can be perceived in a quiet environment. It clearly identifies various characteristics of the problem, but not its cause. Other hearing tests such as word recognition or otoacoustic emission tests (described in Chapters 1 and 2) examine other auditory functions. These tests can in some cases help differentiate the effects of chemicals from the effects of noise, since chemicals might affect more central portions of the auditory system (nerves or nuclei of the central nervous system, the pathways to the brain or in the brain itself). This suggests that the impact of hearing loss on the worker's life may be more pronounced, because not only will sounds be perceived as less loud, but also as distorted. Word recognition may be compromised, particularly in background noise, making it difficult, for instance, to hold a conversation in a busy restaurant or at a party.

Often, it can be challenging to identify the precise cause of a hearing loss. Information on word recognition difficulties or other auditory tests that are inconsistent with pure tone audiometric results can indicate the need for further hearing testing to complement the assessment.

As mentioned earlier, noise exposure can interact with several toxicants. In some cases, a substance will not cause hearing loss by itself, but can exacerbate a hearing loss caused by noise. This process is called *potentiation*. Also, a substance that is ototoxic can interact synergistically with noise, (i.e., the combined biological effect of two hazards is greater than either alone).

Table 6-1 summarizes key descriptors of the effects of the ototoxicants investigated to date. Table 6-2 lists the studied ototoxicants, by class, by the type of possible interaction with noise and sources of exposure. It's important to remember that exposures to these chemicals can occur outside the work environment. Non-occupational exposure can happen from any activities that involve solvents, paint, polyurethanes, paint thinners, degreasers, and fuels.

It's very difficult to predict the exact conditions (such as the exact concentration or period of time) one would need to be exposed to the studied chemicals to suffer an effect. The dose-response lowest observed adverse effect level (LOAEL) and no-observed adverse effect level (NOAEL) have been identified in animal experiments for a few substances. In some cases, chemical exposures increase the adverse effects of noise. Exposures to several stressors, such as physical demands, or smoking can also modify the LOAEL and

---

Descriptors of Ototoxic Effects of Chemicals from Animal Experiments

• Effects observed in different species: rats, mice, guinea pigs, monkeys
• Mainly cochlear lesion
• Medium frequency audiometric range
• Noise exposure not a necessary condition for evaluated solvents, metals or insecticides but necessary for carbon monoxide, hydrogen cyanide or acrylonitrile
• Noise interaction/synergism
• Additive effect between solvents

Descriptors of Ototoxic Effects of Chemicals from Clinical and Field Studies

• Environmental (contaminated water, food or from dust, etc) and occupational exposures to chemicals can affect auditory system
• Auditory effects have been reported following intentional in halation or accidental poisoning
• Increased prevalence of hearing loss as registered in pure tone audiograms (mild to moderate, bilateral, high frequency audiometric loss)
• Interaction with noise not clearly identified as synergist or additive, due to limitations in exposure history ascertainment
• Cochlear and retrocochlear or central lesion sites
• Poorer than expected performance on tests that evaluate more central portions of auditory system

---

Table 6-1: General descriptors of ototoxic effects of chemicals found in the environment from animal experiments, clinical and field studies

NOAEL of the chemical agent. For example, a single exposure to a particular chemical in quiet may not elicit a toxic response, yet, the same exposure in the presence of high-level noise can create a hearing loss (when either alone would not). Moreover, there's a difference in the lowest level necessary to cause an effect in humans and experimental animals. When compared, the levels necessary for an effect seems lower (posing a greater risk) in humans than in animals.

Table 6-2: Substances with ototoxic properties, their interaction with noise and possible sources of exposure

Substance	Interaction with noise	Industrial uses http://hazmap.nlm.nih.gov/
SOLVENTS		
Styrene	Synergism	Manufacture of synthetic rubber, fibreglass reinforced polyester products. Part of floor waxes, polishes, paints, adhesives, metal cleaners and vanishes.
Toluene	Synergism	Solvent carrier in paints, thinners, adhesives, inks, glues, enamels, and component of gasoline. Production, handling and use of toluene and toluene containing products, e.g. chemical laboratory workers, gasoline blenders, lacquer workers, paint and paint thinner makers, petrochemical workers, maintenance workers, painters and printers. One of the 50 most commonly produced industrial chemicals.
Xylenes	No data	Present in motor and aviation fuel, but is also used as solvent in the paint, printing, rubber and leather industries.
Trichloro-ethylene(TCE)	Synergism	Degreaser in metal cleaning operations; in textile cleaning. Also used as a paint stripper, adhesive solvent, ingredient in paints /varnishes, and in manufacture of organic chemicals.
Ethylbenzene	Additive/ Synergism	Unusual in the work environment. As part of mixed xylenes, ethylbenzene is one of many solvents in solvent mixtures (paints, lacquers, rubber/chemical manufacturing industries).
Chlorobenzene	No data	Raw material in chemical synthesis, as a solvent and detergent.
n-Hexane	No data	Production of tires, in glues for the manufacture of leather products and textiles, as a raw material in the production of other chemicals, and as an additive to gasoline.
n-Heptane	No data	Anesthetic, solvent, organic synthesis, preparation of laboratory reagents.
Carbon disulphide	No data	Manufacture of regenerated cellulose rayon (by the viscose process) and cellophane, carbon tetrachloride, the vulcanisation and manufacture of rubber and rubber ac cessories, the production of resins, xanthates, thiocyanates, plywood adhesives, flotation agents, solvent and spinning-solution applications, conversion and processing of hydrocarbons, petroleum-well cleaning, brightening of precious metals in electroplating, rust removal from metals, removal and recovery of metals and other elements from waste water and other media, in refining petroleum jelly and paraffin, and in extracting oil from bones, olives, and rags.

Table continued below

Substance	Interaction with noise	Industrial uses http://hazmap.nlm.nih.gov/
METALS		
Lead	No data	Manufacture of car batteries, sheet metal, pipes, and foil, in mining and in polluted environments. Individuals employed in any of these occupations may bring lead dust on their bodies or clothing into their homes.
Mercury	No data	Present in contaminated air, water, and food, or through the skin. Workers may be exposed to mercury and its compounds in mercury mines and refineries, chemical manufacturing, fluorescent light bulb manufacturing, dental/health fields, fossil fuel power plants, and metal smelting.
Organotins or Trimethyltins	No data	Production of plastics in the chemical industry and as biocides in antifouling boat bottom paints.
ASPHYXIANTS		
Carbon Monoxide	Potentiation	Common contaminant. Product of incomplete combustion of fuels, coal, oil, and wood, also present in gasoline-powered engine exhaust and tobacco smoke. Forging, melting, pouring and welding metals, in farm operations, fire fighting, sewage and water treatment jobs.
Hydrogen Cyanide	Potentiation	Production of acrylic resin plastic, and other organic chemical products, tempering steel, dyeing, explosives, and engraving. Present in vehicle exhaust, in tobacco smoke, and in the smoke of burning nitrogen-containing plastics.
Acrylonitrile	Potentiation	Production of other chemicals such as plastics, synthetic rubber, and acrylic fibres, and is one of the 50 most commonly produced industrial chemicals.
3,3'-Iminodi-propionitrile	No data	No reports on occupational exposures to and no OELs for IDPN were located.
Pesticides	No data	Herbicides, insecticides, fungicides, and fumigants.
Polychlorinated biphenyls (PCBs)	No data	Repair and maintenance of PCB transformers, accidents, fires, or spills involving PCB transformers and older computers and instruments, and disposal of PCB materials. Caulking materials, elastic sealants, and heat insulation have also been known to contain PCBs.

Researchers in France and Denmark have demonstrated in studies with experimental animals that by adding other stressors such as impact noise, carbon monoxide or ensuring that the animals are active during chemical exposure, the lowest level of solvent exposure was reduced before it elicited an auditory effect. This may be true because humans are generally exposed to solvents in combination with a multitude of other factors (several exposures, physical demands, and so forth.) whereas animal experiments typically involve isolated solvent exposures. Another complication in determining the concentration needed for a hearing loss to occur in humans exists because often individuals are not aware of the concentration they've been exposed to, and because many factors can interact in causing an effect. However, unfortunately cases of hearing loss have been observed after exposures that were within permissible limits.

Another challenge in this area is that the number of chemicals studied to date is very small, particularly when one considers the enormous number of existing industrial chemicals and the thousands of new ones placed on the market every year. It's therefore of crucial importance to understand the mechanisms by which chemicals affect the auditory system.

Several different mechanisms can take place and result in an auditory disorder. Some common features can be found between damaging mechanisms resulting from the physical agent (noise) and some of the ototoxic chemicals. A hypothesis is that the damage to the hair cells is caused by the formation of free radicals, so-called reactive oxygen species (ROS). Free radical and reactive oxygen species are ions (very small molecules) that are highly reactive. ROS form as a natural by-product of the normal metabolism of oxygen. During stressful situations ROS levels can increase dramatically, which can result in damage to cell structures. One can be exposed to free radicals through by-products of normal processes that take place in your body, when the body breaks down certain medicines, and through pollutants. The generation of free radicals has been associated with cellular injury in different organ systems. It's considered a basic mechanism of toxicity, and is thought to be part of the mechanism underlying noise-induced hearing loss. Other chemicals such as metals and pesticides may affect both the cochlea and the central auditory pathways, depending on the substance.

When specific ototoxicity information is not available on a particular chemical, individuals concerned about the potential risk factors should look for information on the agent's general toxicity, as well as toxicity related to damage to the kidneys and nerves (nephrotoxicity and neurotoxicity, respectively). Information on whether a chemical produces reactive free radicals could also give some clues about that agent's potential ototoxicity. Glutathione is an important cellular antioxidant that limits cell damage by reactive oxygen species. An antioxidant is a molecule capable of slowing or preventing the oxidation of other molecules (free radicals or reactive oxygen species—ROS). Antioxidants can be used to help treat or prevent some medical conditions, such as coronary artery disease, some cancers, macular degeneration, Alzheimer's disease, and some arthritis-related conditions. Antioxidants include some vitamins (such as vitamins C and E), some minerals (such as selenium), and flavonoids, which are found in plants. The best sources of antioxidants are fruits and vegetables.

Evidence is available indicating that ototoxicity due to noise plus carbon monoxide or hydrogen cyanide exposure (a combustion byproduct) also involves free radicals. For this reason, information on certain chemicals being associated with free radicals or glutathione depletion could also help in the decision to examine a chemical for potential ototoxicity.

Until now few human studies have examined the time necessary for chemical exposures to affect the auditory system, and there is still uncertainty regarding whether it is a chronic or acute process. It is possible that a single, extremely high exposure, as in the case of someone who sniffs glue, will cause hearing loss, as one of the consequences of the abuse. Such high exposures are unlikely to happen in the workplace. Investigations which examined the effects of solvents over time indicated that hearing loss is observable two to three years earlier than is usually seen with noise exposure. Five or more years of noise exposure seem necessary for some individuals to develop hearing loss following occupational exposures. The time needed for a chemical exposure to cause hearing loss is certainly dependent on the specific ototoxicant and the characteristics of the exposure, and needs further investigation.

Considering that environmental and occupational factors other than noise can affect hearing, one needs to rethink which steps can be taken to prevent any hearing disorders. Some of theses steps will be discussed next.

Strategies for Protecting your Hearing
From the Effects of Ototoxic Chemicals

The initial steps of hearing loss prevention programs are hazard assessment and control. It is important to learn if and what hazardous exposures exist in a workplace. Whenever hazardous noise or chemicals exist in the workplace, measures to reduce exposure levels to protect exposed workers and to monitor the effectiveness of these intervention processes are required by law. Some of these requirements are presented in Chapters 1 and 10 and you should become familiar with them. The most effective way to prevent hearing disorders from noise or chemical exposure is to remove the source of hazardous exposures from the workplace, for example, by engineering controls, use of personal protective equipment, or finding alternatives to minimize exposure, (such as reducing the duration of exposure). If the use of personal protective equipment is required, they should be worn as directed. Information on what equipment is adequate for obtaining needed protection can be found at the following two NIOSH URLs:

http://www.cdc.gov/niosh/topics/chemical.html

http://www.cdc.gov/niosh/topics/noise/abouthlp/chooseprotection.htm

Noise regulations pertaining to individuals in the US vary depending on the agency or branch of government having jurisdiction. Among the important ones to know is the level of noise exposure that is permissible. The OSHA Standard for Manufacturing requires that in environments where noise exposure reaches or exceeds 85 dBA workers must be placed in a hearing conservation program. As part of these programs, annual hearing tests are required (http://www.osha.gov/pls/oshaweb/owadisp.show_document?p_table=standards&p_id=9735).

These and other preventive strategies that are used to protect workers from noise exposure will not necessarily protect workers from the effects of chemical exposures. When evidence that chemicals in the workplace can affect hearing is considered, then hearing loss prevention initiatives may be needed even in workplaces where noise exposure does not exceed 85 dBA.

Since 1998, the American Conference of Governmental Industrial Hygienists[1] in its publication includes a note in its Noise Section which states, "In settings where exposure to toluene, lead, manganese or n-butyl alcohol occurs, periodic audiograms are advised and should be carefully reviewed." It also lists other aims to develop specific recommendations and disseminate information addressing hearing loss prevention strategies that are not limited to exposures to excessive noise levels. A similar recommendation can be found in an Australian and New Zealand publication[2] requiring hearing tests for those exposed to ototoxic agents.

Also since 1998, the US Army has added ototoxic chemical exposure to their risk criteria in their hearing conservation program, particularly when in combination with even marginal noise. More recently, the US Army recommends audiometric monitoring for workers whose airborne exposures are at 50% of the most stringent criteria for occupational exposure limits to toluene, xylene, styrene, n-hexane, organic tin, carbon disulfide, mercury, organic lead, hydrogen cyanide, diesel fuel, kerosene fuel, jet fuel, JP-8 fuel, organophosphate pesticides, or chemical warfare nerve agents, regardless of the noise level. The 50% cut-off, while somewhat arbitrary, seems reasonable and may be a good place to start. When dermal exposures to these agents result in a systemic dose equivalent to 50% or more of the occupational exposure limit, yearly audiograms were also recommended. If a worker is currently participating in a hearing conservation program due to excessive noise, the reviewers of the audiometric data were recommended to be alert to possible additive, potentiating, or synergistic effects between the exposure to noise and the chemical substance, and if necessary, suggest reducing the exposure to one or both (http://chppm-www.apgea.army.mil/documents/FACT/51-002-0903.pdf).

Regardless whether hearing tests are offered at work or not, if you suspect a hearing loss, you should see an audiologist. It's important to give information to your audiologist on all exposures that can represent a risk to your hearing.

References

1. *Threshold Limited Values and Biological Exposure Indices* (TLVs® and BEIs®). (1998-1999) American Conference of Governmental Industrial Hygienists (ACGIH), Cincinnati, p. 114.
2. *Australia-New Zealand AS/NZS 1269:2005 Occupational Noise Management/Informative Appendix on Ototoxic Agents.* Standards New Zealand, Wellington: NZ, p. 25.

Suggested Readings

Phaneuf R and Hetu R. (1990) An epidemiological perspective of the causes of hearing loss among industrial workers. *Journal of Oto-laryngology* 19 (1): 31-40.

Morata TC, Franks J and Dunn DE. (1994) Unmet needs in occupational hearing conservation. *The Lancet* 344 (8920): 479.

Fuente A and McPherson B. (2006) Organic solvents and hearing loss: The challenge for audiology. *International Journal of Audiology* 45 (11):367-81.

Morata TC. (2007) Promoting hearing health and the combined risk of noise-induced hearing loss and ototoxicity. *Audiological Medicine* 5 (1): 33–40.

Acknowledgements

This chapter is dedicated to the memory of Dr. Derek E. Dunn

Disclaimer: The findings and conclusions in this chapter are those of the author and do not necessarily represent the views of the National Institute for Occupational Safety and Health.

CHAPTER SEVEN
Tinnitus and Hyperacusis
David M. Baguley, Ph.D.

Dr. Baguley is a Consultant Clinical Scientist at Addenbrooke's Hospital, Cambridge. He studied Psychology and then Audiology at Manchester University and became the Head of the Audiology Department at Cambridge University Hospitals NHS Foundation Trust in 1989. He has over 110 peer-review publications, a Ph.D. from the University of Cambridge, and has peer reviewed manuscripts for many learned journals. Dr. Baguley serves as Professional Advisor to the British Tinnitus Association and holds an East of England Senior Clinical Academic Fellowship. His awards include the International Award of the American Academy of Audiology, the Shapiro Prize of the British Tinnitus Association (twice), and he has delivered the Tondorff Lecture at the International Tinnitus Symposium.

Introduction

It is relatively well established in the public mind that being in the midst of intense sound may lead to tinnitus (ringing), and many high profile musicians are susceptible. One example mentioned in an earlier chapter is The Who's guitarist and songwriter Pete Townshend, who overused headphones at massive intensity while recording in the 1970s and has noise-induced hearing loss and tinnitus as a consequence. Hyperacusis (hypersensitivity of hearing) is given less attention, but can be a debilitating symptom associated with noise exposure.

In this chapter, tinnitus and hyperacusis are defined, and the mechanisms that can cause them to be troublesome as a consequence of noise exposure are discussed. The problems associated with these symptoms, such as anxiety, sleep disturbance and irritability are reviewed, and then hopes for recovery and how this might be achieved through therapy are considered. Finally, prospects for future research are proposed.

Definitions

Tinnitus has been known since ancient times, with references in the early medical texts found on clay tablets in Ancient Babylon, and in medical writings from Ancient Greece and Rome. The word

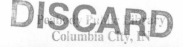

"tinnitus" itself derives from the Latin verb *tinnire* (to ring) though ringing is only one of many manifestations of the symptom. It's worth repeating from Chapter 1 that it is pronounced *TINN'-ih-tuhs* or *tih-NEYE'-tuhs*. A widely used modern definition of tinnitus is, "The conscious expression of a sound that originates in an involuntary manner in the head of its owner, or may appear to him to do so"[1] though even this is not perfect as many people may experience tinnitus that appears to originate outside the head or even elsewhere in the body.

The experience of tinnitus is common. About a third of adults in western countries say they have experienced short-lived spontaneous tinnitus from time to time, and about one in ten says that tinnitus is troublesome for them. About one in twenty adults has sought a medical opinion, and in one in 200 people, tinnitus is severe and has a significant negative impact upon life. Interestingly, if children are asked carefully and in appropriate language about tinnitus, the figures are similar to those in adults. This equates to over 1.5 million Americans having tinnitus that impact upon their quality of life.

Having hyperacusis does not mean that you have supersensitive hearing like Superman. Rather, it describes a symptom where sound that is not especially loud, and not bothersome to other people, seems overwhelming and intense. A scientific definition is, "abnormal lowered tolerance to sound."[2-3] The word hyperacusis entered the medical literature in 1938, but the symptom was not given wide attention until the last decade. Some researchers have made the distinction between hyperacusis and other sound tolerance problems associated with fear (*phonophobia*) or aversion to sound (*misophonia*). A well established self-help resource for hyperacusis called the Hyperacusis Network (www.hyperacusis.net) likes to use the phrase, "collapsed sound tolerance" which carries some emotional impact.

It is not a simple matter to determine how many people have hyperacusis. A Swedish study proposed a figure of 8%, but many experts think this is an overestimate, and the real figure is about 2%. Tinnitus and hyperacusis often occur together: nearly half the people who complain of tinnitus have hyperacusis, and over 80% of people who complain about hyperacusis have tinnitus.

Mechanisms of Tinnitus and Hyperacusis

We have a tremendous amount yet to learn about the mechanisms that underlie tinnitus and hyperacusis, but in recent years some compelling ideas have been put forward. The ignition site of a tinnitus is the point at which it originates in the auditory system. For tinnitus in general, this can be at any point in the hearing system. For tinnitus associated with noise, and in particular where there's a noise-induced hearing loss, the ignition site is very likely to be dysfunction of the hair cell mechanisms in the cochlea (see Chapter 2). The brain does adapt to hearing loss, and that adaptation can also be involved in tinnitus generation. The problem is not limited to the hearing system alone however. There are strong links between areas of the brain associated with hearing, and with those related to reaction and emotion. These account for our ability to be alarmed by sound, and form part of a vigilant danger detection system. The two specific areas of the brain involved in such reactions are the amygdalae (that influences anxiety) and the hippocampus (that's involved in memory). Both have strong links with the hearing system, and the relationship between sound and reaction can be very strong indeed. When a troublesome tinnitus starts, it evokes a reaction as if it were a sign of danger or threat, which can lead to agitation, irritability or distress. There is also an emotional reaction in case of noise-related tinnitus, which can involve anxiety, apprehension, and sometimes fear. This is especially true if the tinnitus is due to trauma (such as artillery during combat), or carelessness by the person or someone else. A vicious circle can then ensue whereby the irritability and anxiety make the person more aware of tinnitus, which in turn makes them more anxious and irritable. For these reasons and more, avoidance of noise that puts you at risk is fundamental to prevention.

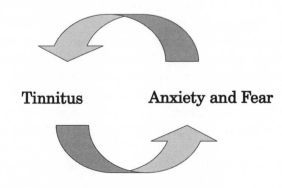

Tinnitus   **Anxiety and Fear**

Figure 7-1: The vicious cycle can be caused by an emotional reaction to tinnitus whereby the irritability and anxiety make people more aware of tinnitus, which in turn makes them more anxious and irritable

Regarding hyperacusis, it should be borne in mind that the loudest sound a normal person can tolerate is about one million times louder than the quietest sound they can detect. This is a fantastic range and is achieved in part by the ability of the hearing system to set its sensitivity depending on how much sound is around it. Another influence is the mood of the person. For instance, if they're anxious, then even quiet sound can seem intrusive and loud. The main mechanism of hyperacusis seems to be increased central sensitivity in the hearing portion of the brain. It has been shown that if people with normal hearing sensitivity wear earplugs 23 hours a day for 2 weeks, then they become much less tolerant to the loudness of sound, a kind of experimentally induced hyperacusis.

Following noise exposure, this sensitivity mechanism can be disrupted so the hearing system is set on sensitive, even when there's quite a lot of sound around. This can lead to hyperacusis, with sound becoming intrusive, seemingly intense and potentially overwhelming. Fear and anxiety may be a consequence of these sensations, and again a vicious circle can make the hyperacusis worse.

It is not just the case that the person is paying more attention to tinnitus, or perceiving the world as louder. In fact, auditory neuroscientists are proposing that areas of the brain actually increase their sensitivity, both to tinnitus (internal noise) and external sound in the environment. This is similar to processes seen in certain types of pain, and is beyond the person's conscious control. Anxiety and fear do have an influence upon this increased sensitivity, and may contribute to maintaining the situation. These physiological insights into tinnitus and hyperacusis are guiding researchers, and hold promise for both better understanding and treatments.

It seems that tinnitus and hyperacusis are linked with each other. If you talk with people with troublesome tinnitus, about 40% experience hyperacusis. Conversely, if you talk with people with a main complaint of hyperacusis, nearly 90% of them have tinnitus. Some researchers believe that hyperacusis is a sign of emerging tinnitus, and some vice versa. The evidence doesn't allow us to be certain about this, but it does seem that the two symptoms are associated.

Problems Associated with Tinnitus and Hyperacusis

When tinnitus is troublesome it can be associated with experiences that reduce the person's quality of life. The first and most common is difficulty with sleep. This may involve the awareness of tinnitus in the quiet of the bedroom preventing the person from dropping off to sleep, or in some people when they've woken in the night, perhaps to visit the bathroom, problems getting back to sleep. It's rare, but not unheard of, for tinnitus to wake people up. Poor sleep can be a significant burden, and among many consequences, can lead to reduced energy during the day. Additionally, being awake in the night and thinking bleak, negative thoughts can potentially lead to low mood or depression.

Another area of concern can be difficulty with concentration. Many tasks in both personal and professional life involve intense concentration, and remembering lists of information. Many people with troublesome tinnitus find that their concentration is reduced, and that if they do have to concentrate intensely for periods of time, this may even make the tinnitus seem worse.

People with troublesome tinnitus may find themselves agitated and irritable, with a restless and uncomfortable energy. This may lead to problems in relationships, and occasionally to people acting out of character in ways they may later regret.

How then is it that the awareness of an internal tinnitus sound can lead to these distressing consequences? This is even more problematic when one considers the scientific finding that the distress caused by tinnitus does not seem to correlate with how loud it seems to be. These apparent paradoxes need some careful thought. The human hearing system is, in part, an early warning danger detection system (as in other mammals). This is why you can wake a sleeping friend by whispering their name, or switching on the light, but waving coffee under their nose might have little or no effect. The awareness and reaction to sound, as with a stalking lioness, is very rapid, and involves alertness, and readiness for action. This is often in addition to apprehension and fear. In this way, a tinnitus signal can become an altering and meaningful sound, evoking lots of attention and agitation. Even worse, a vicious circle can be set up as in Figure 7-1, where the reaction to the tinnitus makes someone more aware of the sound, and then evoking further reaction. It should not surprise us then that a person in this situation may feel restless, agitation and be unable to concentrate. These reactions may be worse in quiet, especially a quiet bedroom at night where restful, refreshing sleep is desired, but unattainable.

The problems associated with hyperacusis are somewhat different. Perceiving the sounds of the world as overwhelmingly intense can lead a person to withdraw and become isolated. Maintaining employment can become difficult, and relationships can suffer when a spouse or a child generates sound that seems painful and intrusive. Behavior can become eccentric; many people with hyperacusis do their shopping late at night to avoid crowds and noise. Some resort to hearing protection (like earplugs or muffs) worn all the time to ward off danger, but this may make things even worse by causing the hearing portion of the brain to turn up internal sensitivity even further as it seeks sound at a normal level.

Habituation can be the Road to Recovery

It is a great shame that when many people consult their physician about tinnitus or hyperacusis they're given negative, misleading, and sometimes incorrect information. This may be along the lines of, "There's nothing that can be done!" or "That'll be with you for life!" Neither of these statements is generally true. The hope for people with tinnitus lies with a phenomenon called *habituation*. This is the process by which repeated and harmless stimulation leads to less and less perception and reaction. This is seen in all organisms from very simple single-celled protozoa to humans. It's the process by which you heard your new refrigerator when you installed it, but haven't heard it since, or when you felt the new shoes on your feet when you first put them on, but now you don't. When you ask people who live next to a busy road or airport how they cope with the sound, they reply, "What sound?" They've habituated to it (grown accustomed to it). This is harder for some to accomplish with tinnitus than with an external sound, especially when the tinnitus is unpleasant and evokes agitation and irritability, in many cases, however, habituation can lead to reduced distress with tinnitus, and sometimes reduced awareness.

This, of course, is less than the ultimate goal of someone with troublesome tinnitus. That is, for the sound to be switched off. This remains outside our grasp, though tremendous research efforts are being undertaken around the world involving drug therapy, and innovative approaches using magnetic and electrical stimulation.

Considering hyperacusis, recovery can be accomplished by the increased sensitivity of the hearing portion of the brain returning to normal. In fact, our hearing sensitivity varies considerably in everyday life, both with the amount of sound around us and our emotional state.

What Therapy is Available?

Until recently, there was a widespread view among both the public and professionals that when it comes to tinnitus, "There's nothing that can be done!" Thankfully, this is incorrect. While it's true that tinnitus cannot be magically suppressed with a pill or surgery, it's also true that therapy can significantly reduce the distress associated with tinnitus, and sometimes reduce the sound itself.

A modern approach to tinnitus therapy first looks at potential causes, and rules out treatable or significant disease. Following a careful and detailed history, and examination of the ears, this will almost certainly involve an audiogram (such as that shown in Chapter 1) and for many people, a Magnetic Resonance Imaging (MRI) scan. Often this will involve a physician or an otolaryngologist (ENT), though an audiologist may take the lead in some parts of the world.

Dr. Einhorn in the next chapter will delve into some of the medical treatments, but if there is no significant or treatable medical condition identified, the tinnitus therapist (usually an audiologist) then explains the situation, often following the framework of:

- Why do you have this (though it may not be possible to be certain)?
- Why is it bothersome?
- What can be done about it?

For many people with tinnitus a careful and detailed explanation along these lines is sufficient for them. In other cases, however, it's clear that further intervention is needed. If issues are identified that fall outside the scope of an audiologist, then some general counseling or specific psychological therapy might be suggested.

Where sleep issues are a concern, some careful attention should be given. The use of simple and inexpensive bedside sound generators has become widespread. These generate a digital recording of rain, ocean, woods and birds to be played quietly at night, but sufficient to reduce awareness of tinnitus. If a partner struggles with the noise, then a special pillow with small embedded speakers focus the sound much more and serves to minimize their partner's awareness of the therapeutic sound.

In even mild hearing loss situations it's possible to utilize hearing aids so that external sound can then be used to reduce the awareness of tinnitus during the day. This can have many benefits, including improved communication, reduced tinnitus awareness, more restful sleep, and less stress. This can be a significant contribution to recovery for many people.

If the vicious circle of tinnitus leading to anxiety leading to tinnitus is evident, some relaxation therapy may help break the cycle. This can be learned from a book, using a CD or by a therapist, depending on the needs of the person. Some clinics use biofeedback to accomplish relaxation.

In some people daytime sound therapy is indicated. This can be achieved informally, with quiet music or environmental noise, or more formally with ear-level sound generators. These devices produce a wideband noise (sounding a little like rain) to reduce the starkness of tinnitus, and other times, reduce the reaction to it. It's recommended that these sound generators be worn at a very low volume setting. Previous advice was to mask out the tinnitus with a louder volume setting and the devices were named "tinnitus maskers." This is an area where sound generator technology has not yet caught up with the digital hearing aid revolution. Sound therapy devices have been very simple, but there are now products that produce digitally shaped sound (including music) and these will be widely available in the future.

Low-level sound generation and counseling are of fundamental importance in therapy for hyperacusis. In this case the aim is to encourage the hearing system to re-establish the usual ability to change sensitivity, thereby reducing anxiety and agitation. Sound is often used to help recalibrate the sensitivity of the hearing system, and some prefer the smoother pink noise* to pure white noise.** What seems to happen is that listening to a sound at a consistent and low level helps the hearing sensitivity mechanism to reset itself back to a normal level over time.

The names given to tinnitus and hyperacusis therapy vary. One well-defined approach is Tinnitus Retraining Therapy that may have the benefit of a cookbook approach, but some find this constraining. The broader concept for this approach is Habituation-Based Therapy, which can include such therapies as tinnitus maskers, Cognitive Behavioral Therapy, Neuromonics, and Progressive Audiologic Tinnitus Management (now used at Veterans Administration hospitals). Even hearing aids fall into habituation therapy because for some people

---

*Random sound whose spectrum level decreases with an increase in frequencies, providing constant energy per octave of bandwidth.
**A sound that contains equal amounts of energy in all frequencies.

they can effectively mask tinnitus. However, there's no conclusive empirical evidence that any of these therapies is any better than another. Most therapists use a general approach and then apply specific aspects to meet the needs of individual patients.

Tinnitus in particular has attracted a vast number of experimental and unorthodox approaches to treatment, perhaps in response to the lack of accessible and effective therapy from mainstream medicine. Examples at present include laser light therapy, and phase-out therapy. Many of these approaches are promulgated and promoted by sincere individuals, though a whiff of snake oil can be detected on occasion. A person with tinnitus can be vulnerable, and disappointment can be an influence in making tinnitus worse. Care should be taken to ensure that any treatment is reputable and has an evidence-based approach.

A Self-Help Approach

While interest in tinnitus has increased over the last decade, some people with troublesome tinnitus may find that there are no professionals in their area with an interest or experience in tinnitus treatment, and they lack the funds to travel to a center of expertise. In such cases one has to look to self-help, not as a last resort, but as a legitimate type of therapy. A first port of call would be the tinnitus societies (see resources at the end of this chapter) that have amassed a tremendous amount of information and expertise. Some areas have local support groups which meet for information and support. Specific to hyperacusis is the Hyperacusis Network, which has a depth of expertise that many professionals would struggle to match.

Sound generating devices are widely available from internet retailers and are inexpensive, as are sound pillows. Some may prefer a CD of the rainforest or the ocean, or recordings of these that are available on internet music sites.

There are also many sources of relaxation, from instructional CDs to yoga and Pilates classes to one-on-one instruction with a physical therapist. A bit of reflection on which route is most likely to suit your personality, and then seeking a source is a good place to start.

As mentioned earlier, for some, the tinnitus and hyperacusis is accompanied by overwhelming anxiety or agitation. In such cases the use of Cognitive Behavioral Therapy can be of benefit, but care should be taken to identify a licensed practitioner.

Themes for Research

Progress in tinnitus and hyperacusis is being made at a very encouraging rate. At the time of this writing, approaches of interest include the application of new drugs for tinnitus (Cambridge and San Francisco) and the use of magnetic (Germany) and electrical (Belgium) stimulation of the brain, all of which seem to hold promise. There is now a community of tinnitus researchers across the world who are communicating and collaborating, with the objective of a deeper understanding of tinnitus and the hope for truly effective therapies.

Summary

Tinnitus and hyperacusis can be unwanted and unpleasant consequences of noise exposure. The mechanisms of tinnitus are not yet entirely understood, but in the case of noise-induced tinnitus, it seems that damage at the level of the cochlea sets up a pattern of spontaneous activity that is sent up to the brain. Reactions and emotions to tinnitus occur as they would for any alarming and alerting sound. In the case of hyperacusis, it seems that the sensitivity of hearing can change, influenced by surrounding sound and emotion. In hyperacusis, sensitivity is set on maximum so that all sound seems loud and overwhelming. Therapy for both involves counseling and the use of low-level sound, often accompanied by relaxation therapy to reduce agitation. In some cases, formal psychological therapy will be needed. Research continues at a fast pace, and experts are optimistic about progress.

References

1. McFadden D. (1982) *Tinnitus: Facts, Theories and Treatments.* Washington, DC: National Academy Press.
2. Baguley DM. (2003) Current perspectives on hyperacusis. *Journal of the Royal Society of Medicine* 96 (12):1-4.
3. Baguley DM and Andersson GA. (2007) *Hyperacusis: Mechanisms, Diagnosis and Therapy.* San Diego: Plural Publishing.

Self-Help Resources

American Tinnitus Association
www.ata.org

British Tinnitus Association
www.tinnitus.org.uk

Hyperacusis Network
www.hyperacusis.net

Acknowledgement

Dr. Baguley's research is supported by an East of England NHS Senior Academic Clinical Fellowship.

CHAPTER EIGHT
The Medical Consequences of Noise
Kenneth Einhorn, M.D.

Dr. Einhorn is currently a board-certified otolaryngologist in private practice in Abington, PA for the past 20 years. He graduated from Georgetown University School of Medicine in 1983 and completed a residency in otolaryngology at Georgetown University in 1989. He currently serves as the Chief of the Division of Otolaryngology at Abington Memorial Hospital. Also he serves as the Otolaryngology Residency Coordinator at Abington and holds a faculty position within the Division of Otolaryngology at Temple University in Philadelphia, PA. In addition to various media appearances, he has written numerous articles and book chapters on the subject of the hearing health dangers of chronic exposure to loud music. He is an active member of the American Academy of Otolaryngology and has served in the past on the national academy's Committee on the Medical Aspects of Noise.

The problem of environmental noise pollution and the health concerns it raises are not new. In fact, in ancient Rome, concern about the noise emitted from the iron clad wheels of wagons clattering against the pavement stones, causing disruption of sleep and annoyance to the Romans, led to the adoption of rules and restrictions. However, the scope and magnitude of the problem pales in comparison to present day. In response to this worldwide epidemic, the World Health Organization (WHO), after several years of work, published their guidelines on noise.[1] This comprehensive report documented seven categories of adverse health consequences of noise pollution in humans.

This chapter will focus on four of these effects as they represent direct, adverse medical conditions that may present to the medical community. These are Noise-Induced Hearing Loss; Sleep Disturbance; Cardiovascular Effects; and Disturbances in Mental Health. Each will be explored in depth as to presenting symptoms, medical evaluation and workup, and treatment options.

Noise-Induced Hearing Loss

Noise-induced hearing loss (NIHL) results from damage to the sensitive structures of our inner ears from exposure to sounds that are either extremely loud or loud sounds over a long duration. The resultant hearing loss may be temporary or permanent, mild to profound in degree, and is cumulative over a lifetime.[2]

While many diseases that affect the human body occur mainly in certain age groups, NIHL crosses all age lines. The Center for Disease Control estimates that 10 million adults in the United States have NIHL, with 70 percent of them under the age of 60. Furthermore, there are 5.2 million children from ages 6 to 19 with hearing loss attributable to loud noise exposure. More than 30 million Americans are exposed to hazardous sound levels on a regular basis. While NIHL is one of the most widespread health concerns in the US, it remains one of the most preventable.

Types of NIHL

There are two types of hearing damage that can occur in the inner ear from loud noise. The first type, as you've previously read, is called *acoustic trauma*, and refers to the sudden, severe, and permanent hearing loss resulting from a single exposure of an extremely intense sound. This is usually caused by an impulse noise (like an explosion or gunshot). The mechanism of injury is felt to be direct physical disruption to the sensory cells of the inner ear.

The second type, known as *chronic NIHL*, is the more common. It refers to the gradual hearing loss that results from chronic loud noise exposure over many years (but not loud enough to cause acoustic trauma).

Early in the disease process, the resultant hearing loss is termed temporary threshold shift (TTS). This refers to hearing loss of brief duration, lasting several hours to days that completely resolves. Irreversible NIHL, termed permanent threshold shift (PTS) may develop after many years of exposure to sounds loud enough to cause TTS.

There are two general theories about the mechanism of injury in NIHL. The first proposes the concept of micro trauma and physical damage to the sensory hair cells and/or their supporting structures. Early on some of this hair cell damage may be reversible, corresponding clinically to TTS. However, eventually the cells are unable to recover and PTS ensues. As it progresses, the sensory cells begin to degenerate and inner ear capillaries can become blocked and collapsed.[3] The second theory attributes the injury to metabolic exhaustion causing progressive accumulation of damaging free radicals and oxidants which, in turn, can lead to cell death.[4]

Symptoms of NIHL

The predominant symptom of NIHL is the difficulty understanding speech (some words are not clear). This, in turn, is caused by hearing loss in the high frequencies. In the early stages, a person may be without symptoms. However, as noise exposure continues and the loss progresses, affected persons may begin to experience difficulty understanding certain words and conversations, especially in the presence of background noise. Distinguishing certain higher frequency consonant sounds (like /s/ or /f/) pose difficulty hearing high-pitched women's and children's voices. Hearing damage in the high frequencies is of particular concern for the musician as it may lead to poor performance, overcompensation, or even music distortion.

Other symptoms associated with NIHL are listed in Table 8-1. They include symptoms that can be just as, if not more, problematic. Two of these (tinnitus and hyperacusis) have already been presented and discussed in Dr. Baguley's Chapter 7.

Symptoms Associated with NIHL

Noise-Induced Hearing Loss: hearing loss caused by sudden or long-term noise exposure

Tinnitus: ringing or buzzing in the ear(s)

Hyperacusis: when sounds that are perceived as loud by most people are perceived as very loud or even painful

Diplacusis: (also known as double hearing) when a single tone is heard as two

Recruitment: when a slight increase in the intensity of sound seems disproportionately greater

Vertigo: an hallucination of motion when no motion is occurring

Dysequilibrium: a sense that one's balance or equilibrium is not functioning properly

---

Table 8-1: Symptoms associated with NIHL

Medical Evaluation of NIHL

The conditions noted in Table 8-1 are some of the most common medical symptoms presenting to an otolaryngologist for evaluation. In obtaining a medical history, questions are directed as to the date of onset, type of onset (sudden or gradual) and subsequent progression (slow or quick). The history should also include questions concerning the presence or absence of other otologic symptoms (ear pain, ear discharge, fullness sensation, and vertigo) which can be indicative of other concurrent otologic diseases. In those patients presenting with tinnitus, it should be determined as to whether the tinnitus is intermittent versus continuous, and pulsing (which we call pulsatile) versus nonpulsatile. As noted, tinnitus associated with NIHL is generally continuous and nonpulsatile. Pulsatile tinnitus may be caused by vascular abnormalities or neoplasms (benign tumors).

Further history inquiry may provide information that may contribute to diagnosis of NIHL (Table 8-2). In particular, noise in conjunction with medications damaging to hearing (ototoxic) has a greater risk of damage than each alone. Some of these medications (like aspirin, quinine, nonsteroidal anti-inflammatories, and loop diuretics) can cause reversible hearing loss while others (aminoglycoside antibiotics and certain chemotherapy drugs) can lead to permanent loss. Smoking and certain common environmental pollutants (carbon monoxide and hydrogen cyanide) are thought to increase the risk of NIHL as well.

Age	
Chemical Agents	Recreational Noise
Pollutants	Loud music
Industrial	Shooting
Diabetes Mellitus	Power tools
Genetic Factors	Motor sports
Genetic Susceptibility	Arcade games
Gender	Risk Factors for CVD
Hyperlipoproteinemia	(Cardiovascular Disease)
Ototoxic Medications	Smoking

Table 8-2: Factors that contribute or predispose to NIHL

Besides knowing about any past otologic diseases, it's extremely important to know about any non-otologic diseases known to cause other types of hearing loss (such as stroke, head trauma, cardiovascular disease, syphilis, acoustic neuroma, severe hypothyroidism, and autoimmune disorders). This also includes tinnitus and hyperacusis (for example, caused by temporomandibular joint syndrome, migraine, Lyme disease, Bell's palsy, vascular abnormalities, and depression).

A general head and neck physical exam is then performed with special attention to the ear exam and, in some instances, the neurologic exam. Laboratory tests may include radiographic exams (MRI and CT scans) and disease-specific blood tests if any of the previously noted diseases are suspected. Audiometric testing (discussed in Chapter 1) and, if indicated, vestibular (balance) function tests are subsequently obtained.

Treatment of NIHL

At this time, there is no accepted medical or surgical cure for NIHL. However, advances in experimental investigations of certain compounds (especially antioxidants) showing the capability of protecting the inner ear against noise-related damage may lead to the development of medications to prevent NIHL in the near future. Until then, besides prevention of noise exposure, treatment includes the use of hearing instruments or aural rehabilitation (learning skills in lipreading and improving innate auditory abilities and listening strategies).

Therefore, the discussion of treatment starts with the discussion of protection. Not only is it important to utilize hearing protection to prevent further damage in the ears of those who have already suffered NIHL, but it is perhaps even more important to target those who have not suffered any damage yet. In keeping with this thought, it's essential that family practitioners and pediatricians as well as otolaryngologists discuss with their young patients the dangers of certain activities that can potentially generate hazardous noise levels (especially loud music, loud machinery, hunting, etc.) and the ways they can protect themselves. The use of hearing protection devices (earplugs and earmuffs) remains the mainstay of protection against NIHL. While standard, one-size-fits-all foam earplugs or premolded earplugs are quite commonplace for most loud noise exposures, these may not be appropriate for other types of exposure, especially music. High-fidelity musician earplugs that do not distort the music quality are now available and can lead to greater acceptance not only among the musician population, but also among those attending concerts and various music clubs.

Of course environmental modifications are another means of protection. In cases where volume can be controlled, it's of extreme importance. I can think of no better application than with the use of one's MP3 player or other personal listening devices. Other types of modifications exist for those in certain workplace environments and for musicians. For those people who are repeatedly exposed to hazardous noise levels, ototoxic medications should be avoided. Also, as part of prevention, medical disorders that contribute or predispose to NIHL should be medically treated.

Medical Treatment of Tinnitus and Hyperacusis

The discussion of the treatment of tinnitus begins with the determination as to whether the tinnitus is severe enough or bothersome enough to warrant medical treatment. For many patients, the understanding as to why it is present and the alleviation of any fears of serious illnesses as well as conservative management are all that is required. Tinnitus severity can be quantified using one of several different, carefully constructed questionnaires. Dr. Baguley presented current nonmedical treatment options for tinnitus in the previous chapter, but some patients require a multimodality approach involving medical intervention for effective management.

Table 8-3 presents some medical and healthcare approaches to tinnitus as well as hyperacusis treatment, but they should be managed by your physician or a knowledgeable healthcare practitioner.

Drug Therapy
- Antidepressants
- Antianxiety agents
- Antihistamines
- Anticonvulsants
- Anesthetics

Homeopathic Therapy
- Niacin
- Histamine
- Ginkgo biloba
- Vitamin B
- Magnesium or Zinc
- Acupuncture

Electrical Stimulation

Temporomandibular Joint (TMJ) Treatment

Table 8-3: Medical and healthcare treatment options for tinnitus

The more common treatments include drug and homeopathy therapies, but their use is much more anecdotal and far less scientific; that is, it's been more a case by case trial and error treatment in the absence of hard scientific evidence.

While there's no medication that has been shown to cure tinnitus or hyperacusis, several have been shown to reduce severity for some patients. It should be noted that all of these medications have varying degrees of success and they all possess side effects (i.e., sedation, dry mouth, and so forth).

Antidepressants, typically the tricyclic antidepressants like nortriptyline and amitriptyline (Elavil), are drugs that do not cure tinnitus, but help treat the depression that often found in severely afflicted patients, thus, enabling them not to dwell on their tinnitus. More recently, flouxetine (Prozac), sertraline (Zoloft), and paroxetine (Paxil) have been used. Antianxiety agents, most commonly alprazolam (Xanax) and diazepam (Valium), initially were thought to effectively manage the anxiety often experienced by tinnitus sufferers. More recent studies indicate that for some (not all) patients the tinnitus itself as well as hyperacusis can be reduced or eliminated.[5]

The anesthetic drug, Lidocaine, has been shown to have some successes in treating tinnitus, but must be given intravenously and has potential side effects. Other medications, including antihistamines (chlorpheniramine and meclizine), anticonvulsants (carbamezapine and phenytoin), and vasoactive medications (histamine) have had sporadic successes, but these are anecdotal and not supported by well controlled studies.

Supplementation of certain vital nutrients and minerals have had limited successes in reducing tinnitus. The B-complex vitamins (thiamine, niacin, vitamin B^{12}, and pyridoxine) are a group of nutrients found in many naturally occurring foods that are involved in many complex body functions that are essential to one's well-being. A few studies have indicated that a deficiency in these vitamins can result in tinnitus. Zinc and calcium are minerals which are involved in transmission of impulses through nerves, including those connecting the inner ear to the brain. Magnesium is essential for certain cellular functions including nerve impulse conduction. In addition to its use for some tinnitus patients, it also has been shown in limited studies to possibly play a role in noise induced hearing loss prevention.[6]

Because of the limited amount of successes and the inherent potential harmful side effects of conventional medications, some have turned to herbal medications to treat their tinnitus. While most of these treatments are not supported by any well controlled scientific studies, many patients suffering terribly with the disabling effects of tinnitus and/or hyperacusis have turned to them when conventional treatments have failed. The most popular herb pertinent to this discussion is Ginkgo biloba which seems to help in increasing body circulation, is inexpensive, and is "relatively" safe. However, for patients with blood circulation disorders, it can function with anticoagulants such as aspirin or ibuprofen to further increase thinning of the blood, so for patients especially under medical care already taking a blood thinner, caution is warranted. Also, pregnant women should avoid its use unless under close medical supervision. That said, it has shown some statistical efficacy in improving the tinnitus for some patients tested; however, the peer-reviewed studies are quite few, most positive claims are from research outside the US, doses are not standardized, and responses have been quite variable.[7]

Electrical stimulation for tinnitus reduction has been used in some form since the1800s. The most popular method utilizes a handheld, low voltage probe pulse system that delivers transcutaneous electrical stimulation at 20 different points around the external ear. These stimulations are often accompanied by relaxation or biofeedback therapy. There is some evidence of as high as a 53% success rate in significantly reducing tinnitus.[7] In the event that temporomandibular joint (TMJ) dysfunction is a factor in causing tinnitus, a knowledgeable dentist or oral surgeon trained in such treatment can actually solve the problem in many cases. TMJ might be suspected when the onset of tinnitus follows dental work.

Sleep Disturbance

Uninterrupted sleep of an adequate duration is essential for maintaining proper physiologic and mental functioning for everybody. While there can be several factors and reasons for disturbed sleep, noise pollution is one of the major causes.

Types and Symptoms of Insomnia

Perhaps the most common sleep problem that noise pollution can lead to is acute insomnia. This condition includes difficulty falling asleep, frequent awakenings, or waking too early. This can lead to alterations in normal sleep stages. Noise can also lead to disturbances of body functions during sleep. These include increased blood pressure, increased heart rate, vasoconstriction, changes in respiration, and cardiac arrhythmias.[8] While this can be detrimental to healthy individuals, it is of particular concern for people with underlying cardiac or respiratory conditions. These effects do not decrease over time.

Secondary effects of insomnia can become evident the following day. These include fatigue, depressed mood and well-being, and decreased daytime performance and alertness.[8] These so-called after-effects have often been cited as reasons for accidents and injuries in the workplace, the home, or on the road.

Noise pollution can also lead to the second type of insomnia, called *chronic insomnia*. That is when symptoms are occurring for at least three nights a week for more than a month. Symptoms include mood changes, deteriorating daytime functioning, adverse work performance, and detrimental effects on one's psychological health. Again, while of concern for all, this is particularly alarming for those with underlying physical or psychological disorders, the elderly, and those with other co-existing sleep disorders.[8]

Medical Evaluation of Insomnia

Ascertaining the amount, type, and intensity of noise exposure during designated sleep hours should be an integral part of the initial evaluation. However, the evaluation should also include inquiry into other causes of insomnia. These are listed in Table 8-4.

The evaluation should also include a sleep history. This will reveal details about one's sleep habits including duration and frequency of the sleep problems, length of time to initially fall asleep and subsequently to fall back to sleep, and the frequency of awakenings during the night. Symptoms to suggest sleep apnea (loud snoring, awakening during the night with gasping and excessive daytime sleepiness) need to be addressed. Finally, other environmental factors (lighting, temperature, TV, or computer distractions) need to be considered.

Physical exam should concentrate on ruling out the various medical conditions that might lead to insomnia. Certain disease-specific blood tests may be ordered.

If an underlying sleep disorder (i.e., obstructive sleep apnea, narcolepsy, etc.) is suspected, an overnight sleep study, called a *polysomnogram*, at a sleep disorders center will be ordered. This test records brain electrical activity, eye movements, heart rate, breathing, muscle activity, blood pressure, and blood oxygen levels.

Psychological Disorders
    Depression
    Anxiety/Stress
    Posttraumatic Stress Syndrome

Neurologic Disorders
    Alzheimer's Disease
    Parkinson's Disease
    Stroke

Other Medical Disorders
    Chronic Pain Disorders
    Arthritis
    Chronic Headache
    Asthma
    Congestive Heart Failure
    Gastrointestinal Disorders
    Sleep Disorders
        Restless Leg Syndrome
        Obstructive Sleep Apnea
Drug Effects
    Caffeine and Other Stimulants
    Tobacco/Nicotine
    Alcohol
    Certain Asthma Medications (Theophylline)
    Decongestants
    Beta Blockers

Table 8-4: Causes of insomnia

Treatment of Insomnia

In the treatment of acute insomnia, it's well-known that lifestyle changes can often alleviate or cure the problem. To this end, if noise exposure is determined to be one of the major causes present, then its elimination is paramount in resolving the condition. Simple measures include closing the bedroom windows, using soft or foam earplugs, or, for some, using a white noise-generating machine at the bedside (a more pleasing sound than extraneous noise). While government regulations of nighttime community noise may eventually be needed, it's beyond the scope of this discussion.

Depending on coexisting factors, several other lifestyle changes can be recommended. These include elimination of caffeine, tobacco, other stimulants, certain medications as previously noted, and alcohol, especially close to bedtime. Establishing good bedtime routines and elimination of distracting visual or temperature stimuli are also important for quality sleep. Cognitive Behavioral Therapy can also be employed to relieve the anxiety and stress associated with chronic insomnia.

Certain prescription medications can be used in the treatment of insomnia unresponsive to lifestyle changes alone. These include drugs that induce sleep (for example, Lunestra,™ Ambien,™ Sonata,™ Rozerem™); drugs that keep you asleep (Lunestra,™ Restoril,™ Ambien CR™); and sedating anti-depressants (amitriptyline, Pamelor,™ Desyril™). Of course, proper medical judgment and guidance is critical as most of these medications can have significant adverse side effects and addicting qualities.

Cardiovascular Effects

A growing number of studies involving workers as well as the general population point to noise pollution as a dangerous and increasing risk factor for cardiovascular disease.

Types of Cardiovascular Effects

The effects can be temporary or permanent. Acute exposure to noise activates the nervous and hormonal systems leading to an increase in blood pressure and heart rate and to constriction of blood vessels. If exposure is temporary, the system usually returns to a more normal state. However, prolonged exposure over time may lead to more permanent conditions, such as reduced blood flow to the heart (ischemic heart disease) and hypertension.[9] Children are also at risk as studies have shown that children living in noisy environments have elevated blood pressures and levels of stress-induced hormones.[10]

Medical Evaluation of Cardiovascular Disease (CVD)

In the initial evaluation, identification of risk factors is extremely important. The more risk factors you have, the greater the likelihood of developing cardiovascular disease (CVD). Decreasing risk factors can help to reduce the risk of CVD as well as the severity of the disease if already present. While there are some risk factors that cannot be changed (for example, advanced age, family history, race, and gender), there are others that can be eliminated, modified, controlled or treated. It's now widely accepted that noise is one of these "modifiable" risk factors. It's important for the physician to know the frequency and duration of one's exposure to noise pollution. Other "modifiable" risk factors include smoking, elevated total cholesterol, LDL cholesterol and triglyceride levels, high blood pressure, diabetes, body weight, diet, amount of exercise, and stress.

Another integral part of the medical evaluation is an inquiry into any symptoms of CVD including angina, shortness of breath, palpitations, a faster heartbeat than normal, weakness, nausea, and sweating. A complete physical exam is performed with attention to sounds of the heart (perhaps listening through a stethoscope), palpation of the pulse, and recording of the blood pressure. Diagnostic tests may be ordered, such as blood tests, EKG, exercise stress tests, cardiac catheterization, and others.

Treatment of CVD

Modifying or eliminating excessive environmental noise exposure (as well as the other risk factors noted) can help to reduce the risk of CVD or its severity, if already present. If lifestyle changes are not enough to control one's heart disease and/or blood pressure, then cardiovascular medications may be added. (The many types and classes of medications used to treat CVD are beyond the scope of this discussion.)

For advanced coronary artery disease, interventional procedures may be undertaken. The most common are the balloon angioplasty and stent and coronary bypass surgery (bypassing blocked coronary arteries with fresh, unclogged, grafted blood vessels).

Disturbances in Mental Health

Mental health is defined as either a state of emotional well-being or an absence of a mental disorder. Noise pollution is not thought to be a cause of mental illness, but it is considered to be an environmental stressor that can trigger the onset of dormant mental disorders.[10] Dr. Bronzaft covers this well in Chapter 3.

Symptoms of Mental Health Disturbances

Studies indicate that environmental noise can either cause or contribute to symptoms which include anxiety, stress, nervous feelings, nausea, headaches, instability, argumentative behavior, sexual impotency, changes in mood, and increase in social conflicts. It can also contribute to such psychiatric disorders as neurosis, psychosis, and hysteria. Some studies seem to indicate that children, the elderly, and those with pre-existing psychiatric disorders (especially depression) may be more vulnerable to these adverse noise effects.[11]

Medical Evaluation of Mental Health Disturbances

If any or all of the previous symptoms are present for any extended period of time, a complete medical history and physical examination is indicated. Questions about noise exposure (as previously discussed) should be asked as well as ascertaining the patient's emotional reaction to its description. History will also reveal if there are any other symptoms of mental illness (such as prolonged sadness, excessive fear, changes in eating or sleep habits, or suicidal thoughts). Other environmental stressors (including death, divorce, change or loss of job, substance abuse,) and indications of past or present psychological trauma should be discussed. The physician may order certain diagnostic tests mainly to rule out physical illnesses that could cause the presenting symptoms.

If there are no physical illnesses diagnosed and the symptoms are significant enough, then a consultation with a psychiatrist or psychologist may be obtained. These specialists utilize specially designed interview and assessment techniques in patient evaluation to achieve their diagnosis.

Treatment of Mental Health Disturbances

Treatment of mental illnesses depends, of course, on the specific disorder, its severity, and its degree of patient disability. Treatment may consist of single or multiple therapies. Therapy options include medications (antidepressants, antianxiety, and antipsychotic drugs), psychotherapy, group therapy, and electroconvulsive shock therapy, among many.

Conclusions

The adverse health effects of noise pollution represent a significant public health concern. It can lead to the development of several physical and mental ailments and exacerbation of various underlying medical conditions. In addition, it can contribute to the impairment of normal social interactions, learning, personal and work performance, and personal safety. What is most disturbing is that this problem knows no age or gender limits and seems to be growing and expanding. Until the time when this crisis abates, it's essential that the medical community take an active role in recognizing the medical consequences of noise pollution, conduct a thorough medical evaluation, institute appropriate treatment when indicated, and, lastly, educate patients as to the potential dangers and means of protection against the harmful effects of noise pollution.

References

1. *Guidelines for Community Noise.* (1999) World Health Organization.
2. National Institutes of Health. (1990) Office of Medical Applications of Research: Consensus conference on noise and hearing loss. *JAMA* 263: 3185-3190.
3. Henderson D and Hamernik R.P. (1995) Biologic basics of noise induce hearing loss. *Occupational Medicine: State of the Art Reviews* 10(3): 513-534.
4. Lynch ED and Kil J. (2005) Compounds for the prevention and treatment of noise induced hearing loss. *Drug Discovery Today* 10(19): 1291-1298.
5. Vernon JA and Meikle MB (2003) Masking devices and alprazolam treatment for tinnitus. In: The Otolaryngology Clinics of North America. Philadelphia: W.B. Saunders, 307-320.
6. Seidman MD and Babu S. (2003) Alternative medications and other treatments for tinnitus: facts from fiction. In: The Otolaryngology Clinics of North America. Philadelphia: W.B. Saunders, 359-381.
7. Steenerson RL and Cronin GW. (2003) Tinnitus reduction using transcutaneous electrical stimulation. In: The Otolaryngology Clinics of North America . Philadelphia : W.B. Saunders, 337-344.
8. World Health Organization. (1999) *WHO Guidelines for Community Noise.* 3.4: 44.

9. World Health Organization. (1999) *WHO Guidelines for Community Noise.* 3.5: 47.
10. World Health Organization. (1999) *WHO Guidelines for Community Noise.* 3.6: 48-49.
11. Babisch W. (2000) Traffic noise and cardiovascular disease: epidemiological review and synthesis. *Noise Health* 2(8):9-32.

CHAPTER NINE

Hearing Health and the Law

Douglas A. Lewis, Ph.D., J.D.

Dr. Lewis is President/CEO of Excalibur Business Consultants, consulting in a wide range of healthcare, business, and legal areas. He is licensed and practices as an attorney, clinical audiologist, nursing home administrator, and insurance broker as well as holding numerous professional certifications in risk management, quality improvement, financial planning, corporate compliance/ethics, neurophysiologic monitoring, and sleep disorders medicine. Doug is a professor teaching for six universities, writes extensively, and is a sought-after speaker in many areas. He is a lifelong musician/composer and continues to routinely "jam" with bands playing a wide range of music—and yes, he wears ear protection!

Introduction

Information and knowledge is a source of power. The goal of this chapter (and book) is to supply you with the basic knowledge and references in the hope of facilitating your ability to seek additional knowledge and information. Hopefully, this will become the basis and rationale for making learned hearing healthcare and other related decisions for yourself.

It is a scientifically proven fact in the biological sciences that deoxyribonucleic acid (DNA) forms the essential building blocks of life. In a similar sense, the institution and implementation of various rules of law are essentially building blocks in the formation of a society. Rules of Law have become the linchpin that often determines how societies are operated and maintained. The mere recognition for the need to have definable laws are essential components in the formulation and establishment of formal bench marks whose adherence to or dismissal of, are used to measure the success or failure of our societies and their members in functioning and acting in an orderly manner.

The intent of this chapter is to aid readers in better understanding the basic foundations, levels, and parameters of law and what potential legal implications or impact hearing healthcare issues may play in the US and other countries. This information is general in nature and presented using a very "broad brush" approach in highlighting and developing interplay between hearing healthcare and the legal arenas. None of the concepts described should be construed as legal advice, but are merely explored with the intent to educate.

Overview

The law has become an everyday part of our lives. One only has to look at the focus various media outlets, businesses and representatives have placed upon issues and proceedings over the last several years. On a virtually daily basis, we're inundated with a multitude of self-proclaimed experts willing to comment upon or directly or indirectly advise the public on the impact or intent of various laws that could or should influence our decision-making processes or actions. Because of the routine media hype various legal issues receive, it would be easy to believe that creating new laws or changing established legal precedents would be a very easy task ("just do it!"—right?). Unfortunately, this belief is a gross oversimplification of an established process and foundation that in some cases has taken hundreds of years (e.g., United States) or even thousands of years (e.g., Europe, Asia) to become established. Most societies over time have created a very intricate process in the formation and implementation of their legal processes and often refer to or include specific document references over time that become the source or foundation for a society's legal and regulatory oversight. The following principles and concepts represent examples of how societies go about establishing the foundation of their respective legal systems.

Hierarchy of Law

Most governments around the world representing themselves as democracies have created some type of document or charter that serves as a "guide" to oversee the affairs of their country. In the US (and many other democratic societies) the document that guides all our legal actions and behaviors is known as the Constitution, described as the "backbone" or "framework" for which all laws and legal actions must conform. If legal actions follow the spirit and intent as elaborated in the Constitution, then all is well and there are no conflicts regarding interpretation and intent. However, if actions possessing issues and considerations involving our legal system occur that are determined to violate the parameters as established by our Constitution, then those actions can be and generally are struck down or disallowed due to being "unconstitutional."

Black's Law Dictionary defines laws as, "A body of rules of action or conduct prescribed by controlling authority, and have binding legal force....It is found in its statutory and constitutional enactments, as interpreted by its courts, and in absence of statute law, in rulings of its courts."[1] Laws may be created and enacted in different ways including statutes, case law and executive order. Statutes are laws created by legislative bodies such as the United States Congress (Senate and House of Representatives) as well as at the state level (Senate and House of Representatives) and local representative bodies (e.g., city councils). Case-made laws are created through adjudication of court cases and the rendering of case decisions within our court systems at the federal, state, and local levels (Appendix 1). Federal law will always "trump" state law or local law (ordinances) when conflicts arise between them resulting in a challenge.

Legal Enactments Impacting Hearing Healthcare in the US

Laws are created for a host of reasons and motivations. Some laws are very broad in scope and are created with the intent to establish formal authority for the government and/or through action of the court system to determine compliance or noncompliance through litigation and other related actions. Other laws are written to enact protections for the public through the creation of government or other nongovernmentally operated agencies to ensure those laws are being enforced and not violated. The following sections briefly highlight just a few of the many enacted laws by the United States and organizations whose laws and regulatory actions may have varying implications for individuals with hearing-related issues.

Environmental Protection Agency (EPA)

The federal EPA was created in 1970 through passage of the National Environmental Policy Act (42 U.S.C.A 4321) which focused upon ensuring all federal agencies study the impact of every legislative program or recommendation that would impact the environment. The EPA became the flagship agency to coordinate governmental actions that impact the environment. These activities include research, monitoring, setting standards, and enforcement. The agency also assists state and local governments along with private and public groups, individual, and educational institutions in supporting antipollution research and activities. While much of the EPA activities have involved environmental and waste product pollution issues, there are increasing considerations to further expand this into dealing with noise pollution issues. The EPA has been instrumental through support of requirements to improve Product Noise Labeling on products made in the United States (40 CFR). Additional research and review is ongoing, but it would not be a surprising trend for the US Government to ultimately expand EPA enforcement activities into active noise abatement efforts through education, training, and mandatory warning labels due to the growing body of evidence of the hazards of high-level noise exposure on the human body (more information in Chapters 1 and 3). Efforts of the EPA were successful in creating the Office of Noise Abatement and Control. This office has no formal enforcement capabilities, but produces considerable public information and advice on the concerns of adverse noise levels. Adequate funding remains a problem at this time, but thirteen states have created noise regulations through these efforts, although the enforcement again remains inconsistent.

Occupational Safety and Health Act of 1970

This act is based on federal law designed to reduce incidences of personal injuries, illnesses, and deaths within the occupational setting. Although all of the parameters of the Act are important, section 5(a)(1) encompasses the General Duty Clause which requires employers to, "Furnish to each of his employees employment and a place of employment which are free from recognized hazards that are causing or are likely to cause death or serious physical harm to his employees." The Occupational Safety and Health Administration (OSHA) is a federal agency in the US created by this Act and was developed to enact occupational safety and health standards and regulations, conduct investigations and inspections to determine compliance with established safety and health regulations, and issue citations and penalties for noncompliance. Twenty-four states along with Puerto Rico and the US Virgin Islands have created OSHA-approved plans at the state level. Most of these plans virtually mirror the federal statutes, but they do permit the entities to adopt their own standards, including the codification of more stringent standards in protection and sanctions than their federal counterpart. OSHA was also instrumental in creating the Occupational Safety and Health Review Commission which is an independent federal agency under the Act that initiates enforcement activities when contested by employees, employers, or their representatives (29 U.S.C.

A. 661). The enactment of OSHA also resulted in the creation of the National Institutes of Occupational Safety and Health (NIOSH). NIOSH is a federal US agency that is part of the Centers for Disease Control (CDC) within the US Department of Health and Human Services (DHHS). The focus of NIOSH is neither regulatory nor in issuing safety and health standards, but instead to conduct research, and develop safety and health regulations with a goal of preventing work-related illnesses and injury (including those potentially due to hearing and hearing loss considerations). NIOSH actively publishes numerous bulletins and alerts, along with creating databases to support these and other research activities.

Noise Control Act of 1972

This is a federal law created shortly after the implementation of OSHA. It gives cities and states the authority and responsibility to regulate noise within their communities. At the time of this writing, over 300 cities and towns have put noise abatement ordinances in place that permit authorities to give citations and render other civil sanctions to those violating local noise standards through their activities. These types of activities are various and far-reaching and include noise from motor vehicles, sound systems, power tools, and so forth. In fact, the state of California alone has over 40 communities who now restrict the use and operation of gas-powered leaf blowers through the enactment of local ordinances protected under this federal statute. The growth of these local restrictions is expected to continue upward as the recognition of the dangers and damage of intense or prolonged noise exposure continues to increase and be realized. Although no formal intensity standards have been enacted on a uniform basis regarding noise abatement, many communities have adopted standards utilizing a maximum sustained intensity level of 60-65 dBA. Additionally, noise levels exceeding these standards are being potentially sanctioned under law.

The Americans with Disabilities Act of 1990 (ADA)

This is a statute that builds upon the antidiscrimination legal mandates implemented by the American Congress in the 1960s and 1970s including Title VII of the 1964 Civil Rights Act, The Age Discrimination in Employment Act of 1967, and the Pregnancy Discrimination Act of 1978. The ADA was specifically created to ensure that "no individual shall be discriminated against on the basis of disability in the full and equal employment of the goods, services, facilities, privileges, advantages, or accommodations of any place or public accommodation." The purpose of the enactment of the ADA was to set guidelines and parameters to:

- provide a clear and *comprehensive national mandate* for the elimination of discrimination v. individuals with disabilities;
- provide clear, strong, consistent, and *enforceable standards* addressing discrimination v. individual with disabilities;
- *ensure the federal government plays a central role in enforcing standards* established in the Act on behalf of individuals with disabilities; and
- *involve the sweep of Congressional authority,* including the power to enforce the 14th Amendment of the US Constitution both federally and at the state level and to regulate commerce in order to address the major areas of discrimination faced daily by people with disabilities.

The ADA is designed to protect against discriminatory practices against individuals possessing disabilities in one or more of the following major life activities:

- Breathing
- Walking
- Learning
- Seeing
- Working
- Caring for oneself; and
- Hearing

The ADA has several subsections to it, but it does address several important hearing considerations in the following manner:

Title I was intended to ensure that people with disabilities have the same opportunities for employment as people without disabilities. Employers with 15 or more employees are required to provide reasonable accommodations to the person with a disability to allow them to perform their job. This law does not ensure jobs, but rather prohibits discrimination in employment for people who are qualified to carry out the "essential" functions of a specific job.

Title II requires that state and local governmental agencies, including transportation programs, make their programs accessible to people with disabilities. Effective communication for deaf and hard-of-hearing people must be ensured and auxiliary aids must be provided. Such telecommunications devices for the deaf (TDDs) include teletypewriters (TTYs) or other text displays; assistive technologies that can include assistive listening systems such as captioning, amplified telephones, and transcription of audio programs. There are also provisions for qualified interpreters.

Title III requires that public places (operated by private entities) including private business, professional offices, and not-for-profit organizations provide communication access. The list of those affected is extensive and includes the following: hotels; restaurants; movie theaters; stadiums, concert hall; retail stores of all types; transportation terminals; museums; libraries; senior centers; sports facilities; and swimming pools. Required accommodations include the aids listed above in Title II as well as television decoders and visual alerting devices (in hotel rooms). The ADA Accessibility Guidelines, first developed by the Access Board in 1991, provided specific requirements for certain accommodations to be provided in new construction and renovation of existing structures (such as assistive listening technology in theaters and other facilities, visual alerting devices in hotel rooms, TDDs, and accessible pay phones in public places).

Title IV requires that all telephone companies provide relay services throughout the United States. Such services must be provided on a 24/7 basis. Individuals may not be charged for such services and there are no restrictions on the length or nature of the calls.

Additional laws that either dovetailed into the parameters of the ADA or were spawned from it that are relevant to both the hearing healthcare provider and consumers of service also include the following:

Hearing Aid Compatibility Act requires that all telephones manufactured after August 16, 1989 be compatible for use with telecoils in hearing aids. The definition of compatible was changed and expanded to include a requirement for a volume control.

Individuals with Disabilities Education (IDEA) requires that children with disabilities be provided with a free and appropriate public education that includes special education and related services to meet the "unique" needs of children. Safeguards were built into the act to allow parents to pursue remedies if their local schools do not meet their child's needs. State and local governments are required to provide education for children through grade 12 in the US and the law applies to public (not private) educational institutions.

Television Decoder Circuitry Act requires all television sets with screens 13 inches or larger, manufactured or imported into the US after July 1, 1993, to be capable of displaying closed-captioned television transmissions.

Rehabilitation Act of 1973 (with subsequent amendments) requires that programs receiving federal funds can be used by people with disabilities, thus the federal government cannot operate in a discriminatory manner. Any grant, loan, or contract to an entity or program, public or private, requires that entity to follow the regulations of the act.

Telecommunications Act of 1996 requires television programming including broadcast, cable and satellite to follow a specific schedule (over a period of eight years and beginning in 1998) for providing captioning. Although there are specific exemptions (e.g., programming shown between 2 a.m. and 6 a.m. local time, programming in languages other than English and Spanish), by the year 2006, all new nonexempt programming must be captioned. This Act also requires telecommunications products and services to be accessible to and usable by people with disabilities, if readily achievable to do so. A major focus of concern for hard-of-hearing and deaf people after passage of this act was digital wireless telephone services, which often interfere with hearing technology and are not compatible with text telephones (TDDs).

Medical Considerations of Noise Exposure

Our world is a noisy place and the types, levels, and intensity of those noises and sounds continue to increase with the expansion of our lives. We are continually exposed to adverse types and levels of noise from a variety of both unwanted and desired sources including industrial and occupational noise, agricultural endeavors, transportation including air, rail, and motor vehicle traffic, music and entertainment activities, social activities in the community (e.g., restaurants, nightclubs, discos), and our general environment. However, the frequency of use and exposure to a number of desired sources such as concerts, music, personalized systems including MP3 players, and cellular phones, continues to increase exponentially as do the numbers of individuals seeking access to these items and venues. A value system that's often perpetuated within our society is that "bigger" or "more" is always better. This attitude is also implied within our acoustic environment and exposure to mean that "louder is better." However, as you have by now learned from this book, medical and health science is showing just the opposite; louder and longer exposures to sound (even wanted or desired sound) can be very risky to one's health and potentially to one's pocketbook! In brief review of some material covered in Chapter 3, there's considerable research to show and confirm that high levels of various types of noise exposure have been directly or indirectly connected to health problems including the following:

- Hearing loss and interruptions with speech communication capabilities
- Tinnitus (ringing or roaring in the ears and head)
- Hypertension (high blood pressure and its effects)
- Vasoconstriction (reduced blood flow)
- Cardiovascular impacts including heart attacks, cardiac arrhythmias, and ischemic heart disease
- Changes in the immune system and birth defects
- Headache
- Fatigue
- Sleep disorders, resting issues, increased body movements in sleep
- Stomach ulcers
- Vertigo and dizziness
- Learning disabilities
- Generalized pain
- Psychological and behavioral stress including increased aggression, depression, and social antisocial behaviors
- Post-work irritability
- Diminished physical and cognitive performance

There is a growing body of legal literature regarding complaints and actions being brought forth as the result of damage to the audiovestibular system from the effects of noise exposure. While many have used these complaints to "augment or support" other claims, there is an increasing number of legal claims being filed where audiovestibular damage incurred from environmental noise is indeed the primary or lead issue. The effects of intractable tinnitus and dizziness/vertigo are pervasive and increasing at an exponential rate with documented cases showing individuals seeking relief by pharmacologically self-medicating or overmedicating, substance abuse, and even suicide! A number of psychological studies have confirmed the deleterious impact high noise levels have upon individuals living near airports, factories, and even within the busy inner city. The number of Workers' Compensation cases being filed due to physical and mental conditions that at least involve some level of overexposure to extremely loud working environments are increasing with many often claiming emotional distress causing psychophysiological symptoms previously noted including immunocompromised body systems, cardiovascular issues, and stomach ulcers. The ability to achieve and maintain adequate sleep because of excessive noise exposure is a growing problem, especially in the achievement of essential Slow Wave Sleep and Rapid Eye Movement (REM) Sleep states necessary for proper physiological and psychological well-being. Although sleep disorders are not recognized under the Americans with Disabilities Act (ADA) as an essential life activity or function (yet!), this author is convinced there is considerable movement toward eventual recognition of inadequate acquisition of sleep being considered as protected due to increasing societal and public policy initiatives. The presence of adverse and/or excessive noise exposure being the "nexus or connection" is one being seriously considered in many legal analyses as viable arguments to support these claims. Hence, the connection of noise to the loss of sleep along with many other psychophysiological anomalies previously noted should not be understated or dismissed within the legal arena and will likely result in further litigation, time and financial expenditures, loss of societal productivity, and a general degradation of quality of life.

Established and ongoing research has diligently affirmed concerns of the previously noted health issues being present within "average" or "normal" populations. However, definitive studies of these impacts upon specific "vulnerable" populations such as the elderly, the very young, and people already possessing certain physical, emotional, or cognitive disabilities are still ongoing and generally incomplete due to difficulty in quantifying and interpreting data. However, it would be easily inferred that the scope and magnitude of the reduced capabilities to cope with adverse impacts of noise exposure would be compounded many times over and would result in members of those vulnerable populations being at even greater risk for the harmful effects of such exposure. I'm convinced that current and future research will support the deleterious influences adverse noise exposures have on our population. Additionally, our most vulnerable members of society will potentially make very compelling and sympathetic plaintiffs in future legal actions. These concerns on their own should be enough to encourage our society to seriously address the concerns of excessive noise exposure through proactive interventions and education at all levels of society.

Noise Standard Study and Establishment

The identified physical, psychological, emotional, and behavioral effects relating to exposure to adverse levels of noise, especially sudden and unexpected levels are impressive and can be frightening. The potential adverse and widespread effects of hearing loss upon the human body appear to increase as our research in this area progresses. The World Health Organization (WHO) has been a highly visible and proactive organization in voicing concerns regarding the potential adverse impacts to noise exposure since the early 1980's. In their 1999 landmark document entitled, "Guidelines for Community Noise," the WHO:

- researched and published their findings regarding specific needs and parameters on how to measure noise
- reported on the adverse physiological and psychological impact of noise upon the human body
- created specific guidelines regarding acceptable levels of noise through the formation of sound emission standards
- reported on how to manage noise issues within our environment, and
- formulated specific conclusions and recommendations regarding their findings along with proposed future research needs.[2]

Their exhaustive work is an eye-opener and has been instrumental in further communicating the serious and profound impact of noise exposures upon our world's inhabitants.

The WHO Community Noise Studies have resulted in the creation of general recommended maximum noise level exposure bench marks with general criteria for various identified environments. A list denoting maximum noise level recommendations as correlated to primary social and dwelling areas is cited at the end of this chapter in Appendix 2. The WHO has also extensively reviewed and studied the potential means of mitigating the adverse impacts of noise exposure. These recommendations include the implementation of various and standard engineering measures, exposure mapping and modeling activities, education and information dissemination parameters, land and facility use planning, and public awareness and efforts to influence noise policy and legislation on a global level.

These legislative and political efforts have begun to show positive impact through the following:

- strengthening noise abatement policies and their applications
- further sharpening of emission standards
- coordination of noise abatement measures with urban planning
- coordination of noise abatement measures and transport planning to specifically reduce mobility of noise emitters, and
- formalized cost/benefit analysis

The efforts of the WHO to inform the public, organizations, and political subdivisions regarding the concerns about adverse noise levels and their impact have not gone unnoticed. In 2007, Neitzel[3] produced an informative survey of activities in various countries in an attempt to mitigate the presence of adverse noise exposure through the setting of maximum allowable noise limits. These limits vary extensively depending on the country. A brief summary of Neitzel's work is found in Appendix 3.

The WHO, OSHA, and many other organizations and entities are embracing established safety and other initiatives in an effort to reduce the impacts and opportunities for deleterious levels of noise exposure. Many of the "Going Green" initiatives often referred to in the popular literature further support these initiatives. Formal hearing conservation programs are now established in the vast majority of entities as the result of formal legislative efforts or by legal and other risk management necessity. These programs constantly identify and monitor adverse noise levels while performing ongoing mitigation activities. Some of these mitigating techniques include the supply and use of standardized or personalized hearing protection devices, the use of acoustic barriers such as silencers, partitions, walls, and tiling to deflect and mute noise exposure, and the never-ending need for viable and comprehensive educational programs for our employers, employees, service payers, governmental and agency officials, legislative representatives, and the public in general.

Potential Legal Implications of Noise-Induced Hearing Loss

Research efforts and analyses have confirmed that hearing loss, environmental conditions, and activities resulting in the exposure to high noise levels have many adverse effects upon humans through various physical, psychological and emotional conditions. Many legislative standards have been enacted with many more standards being recommended. Despite these positive movements, adverse consequences resulting in hearing healthcare issues continue to increase as our environment continues to get louder in spite of the "Green" efforts of many organizations and action groups. Individuals continue to be impaired through actions involving damaging noise exposure. What are the recourses or remedies to this growing problem?

While positive changes are occurring in certain societal values and mores regarding noise reduction, many of these changes are very slow in their implementation and even more in their effect. As a result, those individuals who believe certain protective processes have not taken place, were defective in their construction or were ill-conceived from the beginning often resort to legally-based efforts to seek remedies.

A host of legal actions have been used or can be considered when a perceived hearing injury has occurred. Some of the remedies are obvious while others are perhaps a bit novel. However, they all may represent legitimate concerns and activities and should be viewed as potential legal actions when an injury or deficit has occurred.

There are many laws and agency actions that have been implemented and often mandated as the result of research indicating problematic occupationally related noise environments. Organizations have generally been very amenable in maximizing their efforts to ensure available safety options are in place and generally do this with the best of intentions and in good faith. So what happens when they do not act in such a responsible manner? Organizational insiders such as employees as well as outside contractors and vendors may get directly involved in activities for safety. In the instances of noncompliance, the will and ethical perspectives of the participants are dramatically tested. Proactive organizations should take these differing outlooks seriously and remediate issues where appropriate. When this does not happen, many individuals become "whistleblowers." A whistleblower is a person who alleges misconduct in the workplace. This routinely involves alleged or perceived illegal actions or otherwise unacceptable behaviors such as violations of laws, rules, regulations and/or a direct threat to public interest, such as fraud, health/safety violations, and corruption. They may have to show they're being put under duress to violate standards or threatened in some manner should they not conform to the overseer's improper motivations, (for example, working in a factory and are exposed to noise levels exceeding OSHA standards, and are warned not to complain). There are many reasons that motivate whistleblowers. While most reasons are admirable (like doing the right thing), others may be more personally driven in their motivation (like "sticking it to someone" or financial compensation). Whistleblowers do enjoy some limited legal protections, if their actions fall under federal protection of the Whistleblower Protection Act, The No Fear Act, and the Military Whistleblower Act. Other limited protections include the Sarbanes-Oxley Act, Anti-Kickback Statutes, The False Claims Act, a number of existing state statutes, and any existing company rules or policies. Whatever the motivation, there are considerable risks involved for the whistleblower, such as termination of employment, loss of relationships and affiliations. The primary consideration in the hearing healthcare arena for potential whistleblowing activities are when parameters of hearing conservation programs are not being followed or when they simply do not exist. The parameters are many, but could include such actions as a lack of or insufficient program oversight, monitoring, or compliance, lack of available hearing protective devices, lack of readily available acoustic shielding, or overexposure to adverse sound levels. Whistleblowing could result in various legal remedies such as monetary fines, injunctions or "cease and desist orders." Regardless of the potential options threatened or taken, whistleblowing is a very serious concern and no one should take it lightly. The fact that safety and health are relevant concerns in issues involving hearing impairment alone makes this an addressable concern.

The next area that organizations and individuals must always consider is the area of Tort Law. Torts come in all shapes and sizes with some being considered worse than others. Torts claims are civil court claims and generally don't hold any criminal implications or liability. There are several different categories of torts. The list of Intentional Torts continues to grow as our laws evolve, including those where changes in perceived societal ethical values previously deemed not illegal are perceived as so unethical they should be sanctionable. Some of the more common intentional torts include:

Battery (unwanted physical touching)
Assault (placed in immediate apprehension of injury)
Intentional Infliction of Emotional Distress (intentionally causing some physical or psychophysiological injury through your actions). Some potential examples where these could be claimed might include:

- throwing a firecracker at or near someone with an intent to explode near them that results in hearing loss or other damage;
- horseplay at an industrial site with machinery such as air compressors and nozzles near the ears (This author litigated a case with similar circumstances to this one);
- turning the volume of a piece of equipment up loud so it blasts full when turned on thereby scaring the individual and resulting in some claimed injury; and
- smacking someone hard on their ears with an open palm or cupped hands.

Strict Liability is another type of tort where there is liability without fault and includes:

- *Ultra-hazardous activities* - blasting or other exposure known to cause hearing loss from high intensity sounds.
- *Workers' Compensation* - routine work exposure in loud areas such as factories, flight lines, or the military.
- *Warranties and Representations* - manufacturer warranties or representations that are not followed by the manufacturer or provider on equipment (such as hearing aids, assistive listening devices, or ear-level music players). Reasonable misinterpretation by the

public due to lack of supplied education or information regarding the proper use of equipment or products.

• *Product Liability* - products such as amplification devices or portable ear-level devices that malfunction or are improperly made that result in damage to the hearing mechanism. Lack of manufacturer warnings on the devices may also result in claims of liability from a defective product when some injury or damage is shown.

Negligence encompasses liability from a breach of a defined duty to act within a certain set of standards or parameters and can include the following types:

• *Negligent Infliction of Emotional Distress* - emotional distress resulting from negligent actions by a professional or non-professional where a verifiable injury has occurred, such as a worsening of a hearing loss, or damage to the physical hearing structure causing a verifiable physical injury.

• *Professional Malpractice* - improper or willful negligence from a healthcare professional through deviation of an accepted standard of care resulting in damage or the furthering of damage to the audiovestibular mechanism, such as a ruptured eardrum.

• *General Non-Professional Negligence* - comprises simple or gross negligence. Any action taken outside the professional realm that deviates from those expected of a reasonable person that results in some ascertainable injury or damage. Again horseplay resulting in injury to the ears is common. The failure to supply proper ear protection resulting in damage is an example of negligence. However, if an intent to not properly supply said protection was due to being reckless, willful, wanton, or even a financial basis (didn't want to spend the money) and the lack of supplying it resulted in ascertainable damage to one's hearing, a claim of gross negligence (reckless disregard) would be a potential and valid claim. If gross negligence is proven in court, the civil monetary penalties can be substantial.

Depending upon the scope and severity of the alleged tort, the potential to make inferences and connect tort actions to those much greater could lead one into criminal court if not careful. The difference between them is that a civil wrong is an action brought by one against another whereas a criminal complaint is one brought by a political entity such as the state or federal government against a private person. Both have dramatically different motivations and anticipated remedies. Civil claims often involve the request for a legal remedy such as financial compensation or an injunction (cease and desist order), a request for contract reformation, or other civil process. Criminal claims may involve monetary reimbursement, but are usually also tied to some type of incarceration or significant penalty above and beyond a simple request for financial or injunctive expectations.

One common type of tort possessing potential legal implication involves activities that violate the principles of Strict Liability. These are activities producing liability without fault where one does not have to prove fault, complicity, or negligence. One of the more common legal claims in this area involves Products Liability lawsuits. These often revolve around claims where consumers have claimed injury as the result of a perceived defect of a product. This deficit may emanate from a variety of issues, but could involve such problems as improper packaging, instructions for use, component composition, or output generation (such as electricity or sound). For example, if a toy manufacturer produces and markets a toy gun that emits 122 dB SPL of sound that realistically mimics the real gun's output, there are enormous liability risks to its users and any others around it during operation. MP3/IPod players with no manual or preset limitations to the level of sound/music delivered through insert or other earphones/earbuds may also result in excessive damage to the hearing mechanism. The legal sale of fireworks and related noisemakers emitting excessively loud impact sounds also creates a real risk both to the consumer and to the seller. This becomes an ongoing risk management issue for manufacturers in creating a viable product for consumer use that will indeed be desired and utilized, but at the same time safe for use. Internal process review, assessment, and monitoring are imperative as is proactive identification and action when issues are discovered. Conversely, consumers must be willing and desire to utilize the product and understand that all products generally produce a certain level of inherent risk in their use. Non-meritorious or frivolous complaints can result in unnecessary recalls and/or elimination of products that are otherwise generally considered safe.

Another strict liability consideration potentially resulting from the adverse effects on hearing or related impairments involves claims for potential considerations involving Workers' Compensation programs. These programs have been put in place to specifically ensure that workers are protected from injuries determined to have been sustained in the workplace *regardless* of what happened or who might have been at fault. Being under the auspices of a strict liability standard, Workers' Compensation is a program that employers automatically pay into whether or not they may have claims. There is no provision requiring the determination of fault to be eligible for injury compensation as long as the injury is shown to have resulted from some activity involved in the workplace.

One potential downside for injured workers involves the attempt to bring legal claims against the organization. If they're injured and are participating in the Workers' Compensation Program, they're being compensated for their injury with a goal of making them "whole." Although participation does not preclude an employee from filing other legal claims against the employer, the fact they are already benefiting from participation in the Workers' Compensation Program will be a fact that can be introduced into the proceedings. Many courts are routinely hesitant to further claims they determine will result in a potential windfall for the person filing them who is already fully participating and receiving benefits through programs such as the Workers' Compensation Program.

Another legal consideration that organizations must consider in their interactions with employees sustaining potential injuries or in filing claims involves the concept of negligence. Unlike principles of strict liability, negligence is used to impute or infer liability due to one or more parties being at fault. Negligence generally involves actions that occur as the result of a violation of a standard of expected conduct or care. There are four required elements in a negligence claim; all four elements *must* be met to even have a chance for a successful claim.

The first element involves the rationale of <u>duty</u>. There must be an ascertainable duty to do or not do something. If there is no duty or requirement to perform an action, then one cannot sustain a claim of negligence. The second element involves a <u>breach or violation of an ascertained duty</u>. This may occur in a number of ways. If one has a duty to do or not to do something and they willfully not comply, then there is an obvious breach of that duty. The third essential element of negligence involves <u>causation or nexus.</u> One claiming the occurrence of negligence must prove that the duty and breach of that duty was directly connected to the claimed injury. The fourth element is <u>damages.</u> This is a claim for some type of relief in an attempt to make the claimant or their injury "whole." The concepts of simple and gross negligence play a role in this determination. Simple negligence is not terribly difficult to prove, especially if the duty is ascertainable with an obvious breach and an obvious connection of the injury to that breached duty. Gross negligence comes into play when the action/inaction has resulted in significant injury and the motivation for the negligence was very inappropriate such that the actions were extremely or grossly inadequate, improper, and were such a violation of care that it would "shock the conscience" of even a reasonable person.

One other perhaps more novel legal consideration that hearing and noise issues may trigger is the consideration of a violation of the principle of Quiet Enjoyment. This principle is one primarily found and observed in the area of property law and is not as far of a stretch as one might think. Organizations, property owners, and even tenants should consider this a possible issue when dealing with noise complaints. With the increase in the previously noted environmental issues spawned by increasing noise issues, complaints regarding one's inability under a contract right to be able to enjoy their "quiet and solitude" in their dwelling or occupancy of their land is a type of potential legal risk that could expand into the future and lead to more court-requested claims for relief.

Final Thoughts

It is hoped that this chapter has given the reader some basic ideas regarding the ongoing interaction and in some cases, an inevitable collision between issues involving hearing and the legal arena. The potential for growth in reference to their routine and anticipated future interaction is expanding for many reasons and motivations. The interrelationships are growing as our society evolves and will likely continue to grow with this evolution. Societies that espouse freedom often must deal with these "Clashes of Titans" and the inevitable fallout between the assertion of certain freedoms and expectations with reparations when those freedoms are threatened, impinged upon, or violated.

References

1. Black H. (1990) *Black's Law Dictionary,* St. Paul, Minnesota: West Publishing Company.
2. World Health Organization. WHO Guidelines for Community Noise: http://www.whqlibdoc.who.int/hq1999/a68672.pdf
3. Neitzel R. (2007) Noise Exposure Standards around the World, University of Washington: http://staff.washington.edu/rneitzel/standards.htm

Appendices

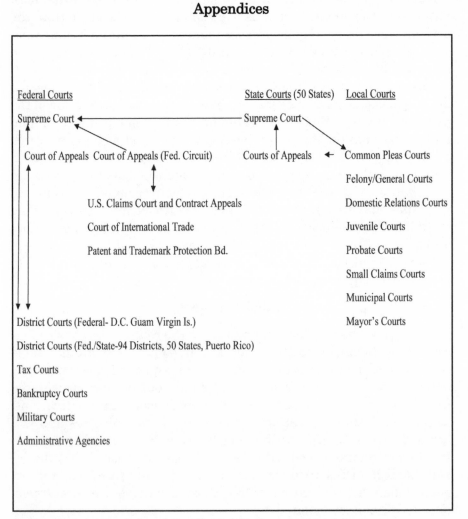

Appendix 9-1: Hierachy of the United States court system

Environments	Recommended Maximum Noise Levels
Hospital and Hotel Rooms and Spaces	30 dB
Indoor Dwellings and Bedrooms	30-35 dB
Outdoor Areas Adjacent to Open Windows	45 dB
Outdoor Activities Areas Including Living	50-55 dB

Areas and Playground*

Industrial, Commercial, and Storage Areas	70 dB
Music Listened Through Head/Ear Phones	85 dB
Public Address Systems Outdoors and Indoors	85 dB
Ceremonies, Festival, Entertainment Events	100 dB

*occurring less than five times annually

Appendix 9-2: WHO recommended maximum noise levels in dBA

Country or Entity	Permissible Maximum Sustained Noise Levels
Argentina	85-90 dB
Australia	85 dB
Canada	85-87 dB
European Union*	80-87 dB
Chile	85 dB
China	70-90 dB
India	90 dB
Israel	85 dB
Japan	85-90 dB
Malaysia	85-90 dB
Norway	55-90 dB
Singapore	85-90 dB
South Africa	85-87 dB
Switzerland	85-87 dB
Thailand	80-90 dB
United States	85-90 dB
Uruguay	90 dB

*The European Union consists of the following queried countries: Austria, Belgium, Cyprus, Czech Republic, Denmark, Estonia, Finland, France, Germany, Greece, Hungary, Ireland, Italy, Latvia, Lithuania, Luxembourg, Malta, Netherlands, Poland, Portugal, Slovakia, Slovenia, Spain, Sweden, and the UK.

Appendix 9-3: Summary of country noise level standards in dBA

CHAPTER TEN

Standards on Occupational Noise Exposure Measurements and Hearing Protectors

Alberto Behar, P. Eng., CIH and Lee Hager

Alberto Behar is a Professional Engineer and Certified Industrial Hygienist. He holds a Diploma in Acoustics from the Imperial College (London, UK, 1971) and has been the recipient of several Fellowships, including one from the Fulbright Commission (USA) and the Hugh Nelson Award of Excellence in Industrial Hygiene (OHAO, Canada). Since 1990, he has been the President of Noise Control and Management consulting company dealing with occupational and environmental noise and vibration as well as with hearing conservation and protection, fields he has been active in for over 40 years. He is Research Associate with the Sensory Communication Group, IBBME, (University of Toronto) and since 2004 Adjunct Assistant Professor at the Department of Public Health Sciences, University of Toronto. Alberto is a chairman and member of CSA and ANSI committees and working groups and is also the Canadian representative at two ISO Working Groups.

Lee Hager brings nearly 20 years of experience to his position as a Hearing Loss Prevention Consultant, including consultation regarding the quality and integrity of hearing conservation programs. He has served as President of the National Hearing Conservation Association (NHCA); chair of the Noise Committee of the American Industrial Hygiene Association (AIHA); NIOSH National Occupational Research Agenda (NORA) Noise Team member; Council for Accreditation in Occupational Hearing Conservation (CAOHC) Council Member; and with ANSI Working Group S12/WG11 on hearing protector evaluation and labeling issues. He presents and publishes regularly on noise and hearing topics, having received the AIHA Noise Committee Outstanding Lecture Award in 2003 and 2008, and NHCA's Threadgill Award for service in 2004.

Introduction

Standards try to help manage the world we live in and the things we do in a manner that is repeatable and manageable. The standards process ensures that when we buy a pound of coffee, it's really a pound, and that a quart of milk is really a quart. People sometimes ask, what are standards? Why do we need them? Who writes them, and who's responsible for publishing them and keeping them up to date?

What are Standards?

Wikipedia, the free encyclopedia (http://www.wikipedia.org) states that a technical standard is, "...an established norm or requirement." It's usually a formal written document that establishes uniform engineering or technical criteria, methods, processes and practices.

Standards are "best practices" that describe how to consistently do important things in a way that is understood and repeatable—things like electrical standards, for example, describe how houses are to be wired (so the electrician knows which wire is which) and what is meant by "117V AC" (so the microwave manufacturer puts the right parts inside their appliance).

Standards essentially provide specifications and descriptions about "how to." Most often they deal with how to measure, or how to build or, finally, how to manage. In this chapter, the standards of interest describe how to measure workplace noise exposure, how to estimate the effect of noise exposure on one's hearing, and how to determine the effectiveness of hearing protectors.

Some standards go beyond measuring, and describe how to apply information. The hearing protector evaluation standards described here provide such an example. Some standards also provide direct guidance to end users, for example, on how to select appropriate hearing protection devices for certain kinds of noise levels, or how to use and care for these devices.

It's important to recognize that standards development is an ongoing process. The people who develop standards are constantly working to improve and update these documents to reflect new scientific findings, new technologies, or improved practices in their areas of interest. The standards discussed in this chapter may undergo revision at any time, and the reader is encouraged to investigate the most recent revision for the latest information.

How are Standards Developed?

Experts in a given field determine that there is a need to establish a "norm" or standard practice. This might be a need to conduct some activity consistently and reliably, so that when this activity is done by different groups of people, (within the same or different countries) the results from each group can be compared "apples-to-apples." It may be a need to specify important guidelines, such as how loud emergency warning signals should be in offices as opposed to manufacturing environments. The experts decide when it's time to develop a standard.

Standards are typically developed by groups of subject matter experts (SMEs). These are people with specific expertise on the topic of interest. Most standards development committees (in the US, these are referred to as "Working Groups") are ad hoc, meaning that they assemble to write a particular standard on a specific topic. Experts are volunteers and work on an honorarium basis (unpaid). Once the standard has been approved, the SME may be dissolved and assembled again either for a revision or for writing another standard on the same topic. Decisions within the committee are typically determined by consensus, so that everyone working on the standard must agree on what is finally written.

Once a draft standard is prepared by the committee, it's sent for review and/or discussion to interested parties. These may be people who the proposed standard may affect, but who may not have the specific expertise or interest to work on developing the standard. For example, not all manufacturers who make noise in their plants may have the time or interest to participate in the time-consuming process of developing a standard on hearing protectors, but the final standard will certainly affect them. Nevertheless, they or their representatives (such as industry-specific manufacturing associations or trade groups) have a say in what the final document looks like. These groups may participate in the review, but not necessarily in the development of the standard.

Comments from reviewers are taken seriously and must be resolved by the standards development committee before the standard can go any further in the process. After reviewer comments are addressed and resolved, the standard is formatted and circulated for a final review. Only after this extensive review and approval process can the standard finally be published. They are then sold by the standards oversight institutions to defray some of the costs of standard development activity.

Standards are reviewed periodically, usually every 5 years. Subject matter experts (SMEs) consider new scientific developments in the field, new technologies, the applicability of the standard and their technical aspects, and how the standard has been used by end users. The SMEs may then simply re-approve the standard as is, make small changes, or undertake a wholesale revision of the standard as they deem appropriate.

Standards are developed both on a national basis as well as internationally. National standards are typically developed to address the specific needs of each county, while international standards are adopted in areas where cross-border cooperation is crucial (such as the European Union) or where local, national standards do not exist. International standards are written also by experts that belong in many cases to their local standards institutions. That's why often the standards developed nationally are very similar to international standards and vice versa. Efforts are made to "harmonize" national and international standards to level the playing field globally.

How are Standards Used?

Standards are used (in our case) to ensure that everyone who is in the business of measuring noise exposure or hearing protector performance will do it in the same way so that the test results they get are consistent. In other words, the results of the measurements should be comparable across measuring laboratories, across individuals wearing protectors, and among people who measure noise exposure levels. The same hearing protector measured in different laboratories should show about equal levels of protection, and the same noise conditions should give the same exposure results regardless of where and who is doing the measurement.

Standards are not regulations and are not enforceable as such. They're consensus efforts that describe the best knowledge and science at the time they were developed, as interpreted by the SMEs. Standards are often referred to in regulations, and serve as the technical basis for most regulations, but are not laws in and of themselves. For example, in the US, the federal government has issued a law (the US Hearing Conservation Amendment, 29 CFR 1910.95) that regulates the amount of noise a worker may be exposed to, and the protective actions necessary when noise exceeds critical levels. This law refers to a number of different standards addressing different issues.

- Allowable background sound levels in hearing testing environments (ANSI S3.1)
- Hearing test equipment (ANSI S3.6)
- Noise measurement equipment (ANSI S1.4 and S1.25)

So the standards process informs and supports regulations without being regulatory itself.

Who Develops Standards?

SMEs are drawn from groups with specific interest and expertise in the area addressed by the standard, such as governmental institutions, end users and manufacturers. These experts are non-paid volunteers who meet to discuss and debate the different issues involved with each topic area and come to consensus about the best way to approach them.

Standards development committees are nongovernment bodies kept at arm's length from each government to insure total independence. They're responsible to national or international standards management groups, who publish and distribute the standards developed by the committee.

Here we will be dealing with three standard institutions only:

- the Canadian Standards Association (CSA)
  www.csa.ca/Default.asp?language=english
- the American National Standards Institute (ANSI)
  www.ansi.org
- the International Standards Organization (ISO)
  www.iso.org/iso/home.htm

How are Standards Organized?

Canadian Occupational Health and Safety (OHS) standards are provided in the following areas:
(http://ohs.csa.ca/standards/index.asp)

- Construction Safety
- Electrical
- Emergency Preparedness
- Equipment & Machinery Safety
- Ergonomics / Human Factors
- General Workplace Safety
- OHS Management Systems
- Personal Protective Equipment

Hearing protectors are included in the Personal Protective Equipment area, and noise and hearing measurement are addressed in the General Workplace Safety area under Acoustics and Noise Control. On the other hand, the Noise Exposure Standard is the responsibility of the Acoustics and Noise Control group.

ANSI standards are organized by topic area, with Accredited Standards Committee S1 dealing with Acoustics, S2 handling Mechanical Vibration and Shock, S3 on Bioacoustics, and S12 Noise. The Acoustical Society of America is the "secretary" of noise and hearing-related standards in the US. Complete lists of US acoustics related standards (http://asa.aip.org/standards/NatCat.pdf) as well as standards developed in conjunction with international partners (http://asa.aip.org/standards/IntnatCat.pdf) are available from ASA.

Each ANSI standard is identified with a combination of numbers and letters that describe a range of things about the standard. For example, ANSI/ASA S1.1-1994(R2004) indicates it:

- is an American national standard (ANSI) managed by the Acoustical Society of America (ASA)
- pertains to acoustics (S)
- is managed by the S1 Acoustics committee (1)
- is their first standard (.1)
- last underwent major revision in 1994 (-1994)
- underwent minor revision and reaffirmation in 2004 (R2004)

ISO standards pertaining to noise and hearing are managed by Technical Committee (TC) 43, Subcommittee (SC) 1 (www.iso.org/iso/iso_catalogue/catalogue_tc). While ISO uses a different standards cataloguing/numbering system than CSA or ANSI, the topic descriptions make it easy to find standards of interest.

Hearing Protector Standards

Hearing protector standards can be divided into three groups. Measurement Standards - techniques for assessing how well hearing protectors work, both in the laboratory and in actual use. Applications Standards - how to apply the results of measurements to estimate how well hearing protectors might actually work for people using them in real world situations. Combination Standards - techniques for both of these applications.

Hearing Protector Measurement Standards

The most common way to assess how well hearing protectors work is called the *real-ear attenuation at threshold* (REAT) test. This approach uses human test subjects, and tries to measure the quietest sound they can reliably hear at a range of different frequencies or tones, from low-pitched, "boomy" tones to high-pitched, hissing sounds. This "just detectable" sound level is called the *threshold of hearing*.

The threshold is measured without the hearing protector, then again with the hearing protector in place. The difference between these two sets of hearing test measurements reflects the effective reduction in noise provided by the hearing protector, known as *attenuation*. The attenuation is specific to that particular protector, that individual, that frequency and that test.

Measurement standards describe how to conduct these tests and how to use REAT testing to estimate attenuation. Testing is done in a specified acoustic environment with test signals covering the whole range of tones that humans can typically hear. This environment is actually a semi-anechoic room. That is, it's a very well-insulated enclosure from the exterior noise where almost all acoustic energy is absorbed, resulting in very little acoustic reflections and almost no echo. In this room, the audible frequencies run the range from very low tones (125 Hz) to very high tones (8000 Hz). For comparison, the frequency of middle C on a piano is 262 Hz, and each doubling of frequency (for example from 125 Hz to 250 Hz) yields a tone that is one octave higher.

Groups of test subjects (either 10 or 20 depending on the hearing protector to be tested) are used, and multiple tests are conducted on each person. All of this information is statistically analyzed and averaged (with safety factors) to estimate the range of attenuation of a given hearing protector. As you can imagine whenever people are involved there are sometimes issues of test-retest reliability. Part of the testing involves measuring the extent of this reliability and is typically summarized by the statistical term "standard deviation" or "variance."

The Standards

The following are measurement standards:
1. ANSI/ASA S12.6-2008: *American National Standard Methods for Measuring the Real-Ear Attenuation of Hearing Protectors*

This standard specifies laboratory-based procedures for measuring, analyzing, and reporting the noise-reducing capabilities of hearing protection devices. It includes both a process that uses well-trained human subjects called Method A as well as a process that uses inexperienced subjects called Method B. The primary difference between these is that under Method A, subjects are fully trained as to the use of the hearing protector being tested. They're given lots of opportunity to practice using the protectors, and lots of coaching by the person doing the test to make sure the protectors are used correctly. By contrast, in Method B, test subjects are people who have very limited or no experience in using hearing protectors, and the only guidance they receive for using the hearing protectors are the instructions printed on the hearing protectors' packaging.

Method A is a good reflection of how much protection may be provided in ideal conditions or how much protection the device is capable of providing if used perfectly, where Method B may be a more realistic assessment of how hearing protectors are used in the real world and the amount of protection most users could expect to get.

2. ISO 4869-1:1990: *Acoustics - Hearing protectors - Part 1: Subjective method for the measurement of sound attenuation,* and ISO/TS 4869-5:2006: *Acoustics - Hearing protectors - Part 5: Method for estimation of noise reduction using fitting by inexperienced test subject*
These are international versions of ANSI/ASA S12.6-2008. While there are small differences between the ANSI and ISO standards, they're not significant. ISO has placed the trained-subject and inexperienced-subject protocols into different standards.

3. ISO 4869-3:2007 *Acoustics - Hearing protectors - Part 3: Measurement of insertion loss of earmuff type protectors using an acoustic test fixture* and ANSI S12.42-1995 (R2004) *American National Standard Microphone-in-Real-Ear and Acoustic Test Fixture Methods for the Measurement of Insertion Loss of Circumaural Hearing Protection Devices.*
These standards describe a different approach to measuring hearing protector performance. They specify how to use acoustical test fixtures (ATF) in place of human subjects to test certain hearing protectors. ATFs, also known as *artificial heads* or *acoustic manikins,* contain microphones located inside the "head." This allows measurement of sounds levels outside and inside the ATF, with and without the hearing protector in place, reflecting a direct measure-

ment of protection when the hearing protector is donned.

While it may seem like the ATF approach would be the best way to test hearing protectors, experience has shown that using real people as test subjects gives a better sense of how well hearing protectors really work in the real world. The variability among the sizes and shapes of peoples' ear canals and the differing ability of people to use the devices affect the fit, and therefore the ultimate performance, of hearing protectors. Capturing this variability by using a more or less random group of human subjects makes REAT testing the preferred approach in most situations. However, in some situations, such as research and development of new hearing protectors, or in conditions where the noise levels used for testing may be dangerous to human subjects, the ATF can provide a good and safe substitute.

4. ISO/TR 4869-4:1998 ISO *Acoustics - Hearing protectors - Part 4: Measurement of effective sound pressure levels for level-dependent sound-restoration earmuffs* addresses a specific type of hearing protector.

This standard describes a way to test specialized hearing protectors (primarily earmuffs) that have microphone(s) on the outside that allow some environmental sounds to pass through. Those sounds are fed into electronic circuits inside the earmuff and play through a small loudspeaker inside the protector. The transfer electronics are selective and keep sound levels safe by limiting the sounds passed through to less than a given limit (typically 82 dBA to 85 dBA). Those protectors are useful in situations where the noise level is moderate or intermittent, but may on occasion exceed the 85 dBA "safe" limit. Amplifying the sound improves intelligibility of speech when the hearing protector is used.

Hearing Protector Measurement Application Standards

These standards describe how to use the results of the measurements collected using the standards described previously (typically laboratory-based measurements) to estimate the protection provided by hearing protectors in actual use by actual people in actual noise. Translation of laboratory findings to real world attenuation can be challenging, given the amount of variability in hearing protector performance.

It's also important to keep in mind that the precision of the estimates that come from the standards presented next will be driven in large part by the amount, accuracy, and format of noise exposure information. Keeping this information linked is one of the keys to preventing hearing loss in noise.

1. ISO 4869-2/Cor1:2006 *Acoustics - Hearing protectors - Part 2: Estimation of effective A-weighted sound pressure levels when hearing protectors are worn.*

This standard describes three different ways to estimate this assessment, each with a different level of precision. The simplest approach uses a single number estimate of attenuation as derived from the standards just described, subtracted from the noise exposure level measured in C-weighted decibels (dBC). (The dBC or C-weighted noise level is simply the actual measurement with a sound level meter without any corrections for "how the ear hears" as would be the case with dBA or A-weighted noise levels). This approach is easiest to use, but less accurate than the other methods described in this standard.

A second approach provides a calculation that limits the result to only three numbers in different tonal or frequency ranges that have to be combined to obtain the desired outcome. Instead of one attenuation number, attenuation is calculated for a range of low, middle and high tones, and the protection in each frequency range can be subtracted from the noise exposure in each range to estimate the amount of noise getting through to the person using the hearing protector.

The most precise approach requires the measurement of noise exposure in octave bands, meaning a separate value for each range of frequencies in the exposure from low to high tones. This kind of information is not normally collected during a noise survey, so typically this application is only used in special situations.

2. ANSI/ASA S12.68-2007 *Methods of Estimating Effective A-Weighted Sound Pressure Levels When Hearing Protectors are Worn.*

This Standard includes an approach similar to the octave band method just described (the second approach in ISO 4869-2/Cor1: 2006). In addition, it provides two other approaches with procedures for the calculation of two different estimates to be subtracted from the noise exposure level measured in either dBC or A-weighted decibels (dBA) or a comparison of both.

Each estimate predicts the attenuation that a given percentage of users will receive, typically from the upper 20% (an estimate of the most motivated and best protected users of the hearing protector) to the upper 80% (an estimate of the amount of protection most users should be able to get with a reasonable amount of training). Providing attenuation estimates in this manner helps users understand that a range of performance is to be expected from a given hearing protector. It enables people purchasing and distributing hearing protectors in the workplace to select appropriate devices based on their knowledge and understanding of noise-exposed workers and their hearing protector use habits and patterns.

Combination Standard

This is a standard that deals with both measurement and usage: CAN/CSA-Z94.2-02 (R2007): *Hearing Protection Devices - Performance, Selection, Care, and Use.*

This standard describes how to select which hearing protectors may be appropriate for given noise exposure levels. It is intended to guide manufacturers as to how to label their devices, and users in making appropriate selection of hearing protectors.

It specifies that attenuation should be measured following ANSI/ASA S12.6-2008 and proposes two ways of calculating the net effectiveness of the hearing protector as reflected by the noise level reaching the protected ear using different estimates. This standard also contains an extensive section for the user that includes information and orientation regarding the selection, care and use of the hearing protectors as well as information regarding some non-traditional protectors, their usage and application.

Noise Exposure Measurement Standards

These standards describe techniques for gathering noise exposure information and processes for analyzing and interpreting the information collected. Standards also have been written on a range of related topics, including accuracy of noise measurement equipment, but here we'll address only those standards dealing with workplace noise measurement.

1. ANSI S12.19-1996 (R2006) *American National Standard Measurement of Occupational Noise Exposure*
This standard describes how to effectively use a range of noise measurement instruments which include:

- sound level meters (SLMs) that provide instantaneous reading of noise level (see Figure 1-2, Page 7);

- integrating sounds level meters (ISLMs) that
  average sound levels over time; and

- dosimeters that are designed to be worn by a worker
  for an extended period of time to average personal
  noise exposure in order to assess the amount of noise
  people are exposed to on the job (see Figure 1-3, p.14)

This standard does not describe any limits to exposure or provide
any guidance as to what to do with the measurements. It simply describes how to use each instrument effectively.

2. CSA Z107.56-06: *Procedures for the measurement of occupational
noise exposure*
Guidance is provided here to help in appropriate selection of instruments (SLMs and/or noise dosimeters) and procedures for measurement in different kinds of noise environments. It provides
statistical support on how to analyze data to estimate noise exposure
for groups of workers by measuring a limited number of subjects. It
also emphasizes the importance of subject cooperation with noise
measurement processes and a number of other practical tools to help
in noise measurement projects.

3. ANSI S3.44-1996 (R2006): *Determination of occupational noise
exposure and determination of noise-induced hearing impairment*
While this standard describes how to apply information collected
in accordance with ANSI S12.19-1996 (R2006) to estimate noise
exposure, it also estimates the effect of that noise exposure on people.
By looking at noise exposure over time, this standard provides estimates of the damage to hearing that could be expected at a range of
susceptibility levels, from the 10% most susceptible to the 90% least
susceptible.

4. ISO 9612:2009(E): *Determination of occupational noise exposure-
Engineering method*
Depending on the situation, this standard describes a range of
different approaches to collecting noise exposure information, from
measurement of task-related noise and extrapolation to full days, to
full day measurements, to full day projections based on task-level
measurement and task-duration information. It provides guidance
on which approach is best, how many measurements are necessary

for reliability, and how to analyze information to draw the best conclusions about long-term risk of noise exposure.

ISO 9612 also includes a discussion about uncertainty. That is, what things may factor into decisions about how reliable the data actually are.

Conclusion

Standards are useful tools to help ensure reliability and consistency in noise exposure assessment and hearing protector performance. Look to make sure that the hearing protectors you use are tested to the appropriate standard, and make sure that noise exposure information, combined with the hearing protectors' attenuations meet the appropriate criteria to prevent occupational hearing loss.

CHAPTER ELEVEN
Architectural Strategies to Minimize Noise
William J. Gastmeier, MASc. PEng.

Bill Gastmeier is a principal partner of HGC Engineering, a consulting engineering firm specializing in Acoustics, Noise and Vibration. He has more than 30 years of professional experience in Acoustical Engineering having graduated with an undergraduate degree in Honours Physics (1974) and a Masters Degree in Electrical Engineering (Acoustics, 1976) from the University of Waterloo. He is a Registered Professional Engineer and a Designated Consulting Engineer in the Province of Ontario, a member of the Acoustical Society of America (ASA) and the Canadian Acoustical Association (CAA). He holds several US Patents in Acoustics and is an Adjunct Professor in the School of Architecture at the University of Waterloo and a lecturer in Acoustics at Dalhousie University in Halifax.

Introduction

A very effective way to minimize noise is to control it at the source, or "Turn down the volume!" Not unexpectedly, some noise sources are easier to control than others, or are outside the control of the person receiving the noise, so simply turning it down is not always possible. In this chapter we examine ways to control noise along the path of its transmission where a wide variety of means are available, often involving the architecture of the spaces in which we live, work and play.

Source—Path—Receiver

In any real acoustical situation there are three basic elements to consider (shown in Figure 11-1).
1) The sound source (which can be desirable or undesirable).
2) The path for the transmission of sound.
3) The receiver who may or may not want to listen to the sound.

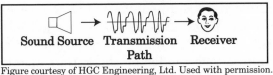

Figure courtesy of HGC Engineering, Ltd. Used with permission.

Figure 11-1: Source—path—receiver

If the sound is desirable, favorable conditions are provided for its production, transmission and reception. In a theater or worship space the talker is elevated on a stage or platform with respect to the listener. The transmission path (air) is made more effective by the use of reflective surfaces or a sound system, and thus, the receiver is provided with excellent listening conditions.

If the sound is undesirable such as noise from a neighbor's television set or noise from machines in a workplace, for example, conditions may still exist for its production, transmission and reception. However, measures can be taken to suppress the noise at the source. The effectiveness of the transmission path can be reduced, often by use of partitions, barriers or enclosures that are adequately soundproofed. Thereby, the people subjected to the cacophony are protected or made tolerant of the disturbance.

Sound Power and Sound Pressure

It is helpful here to introduce the concept of sound power and differentiate it from the concept of sound pressure discussed in previous chapters. The Sound Power Level (sometimes written as Lw) is the amount of sound in decibels emitted by a source and is the more basic quantification of sound. It's specific to the source and is not dependent on the nearby environment. The Sound Pressure Level (sometimes written as SPL or Lp) in decibels, on the other hand, is the response of the transmission medium (air) to the emitted sound power. Sound pressure is what we hear, and it depends strongly on the environment.

There is a close analogy with the use of an electric heater. The heater produces a specific amount of power that does not change (unless you turn it down) and the resulting temperature in the room varies with many factors such as location, distance, insulation in the walls, and the presence of openings, such as windows.

The first step in controlling noise is to know how much sound power the noise source produces. However, in the US, noise labeling at the present time is only voluntary. Recent efforts at standardization have provided the tools to accurately measure and label the sound power emitted by equipment used in the workplace and appliances used in the home. Buyers—both residential and commercial—should look for products that have noise labels if available. This is a great advantage over older methods that usually referred to noise emissions using qualitative terms. Think of the "whisper quiet" dishwasher that sounds more like a jet engine with a "Hush Kit" when you're trying to sleep. In fact, dishwashers are a consumer appliance which most manufacturers label with the noise emission rating.

Sound power is also rated in A-weighted decibels (dBA), discussed in earlier chapters, so it's important to know which quantity, sound power (Lw) or sound pressure (SPL or Lp) is referred to in a particular instance. The advantage is that you know if you purchase equipment with a lower sound power value on the label, it really will be quieter than equipment with a higher rating, not withstanding all the environmental conditions that affect sound pressure, as discussed next. This is the first step in the design of quieter workplaces. Through acoustical engineering methods the sound power value can be used to accurately calculate the sound pressure that will be present at different locations in a room or workplace before the space is built or the machine is installed, and thereby design workplaces that are more hearing friendly.

Factors Affecting the Distribution of Sound Pressure in a Room

1. Source Directivity

All sound sources other than a pulsating sphere have a certain amount of directionality or directivity. That is, they radiate sound more effectively in one direction than in another. An important example of this is the human voice. It's much easier for someone to hear you if you are facing directly toward them. This is especially important when you're speaking to someone with a hearing loss. So a solution in communication is to be aware of directivity and manipulate the environment to your advantage.

The voice is most directional for the higher frequency consonants that are most important for intelligibility. It's the least directional for the lower frequency vowel sounds, as shown in Figure 11-2. If one

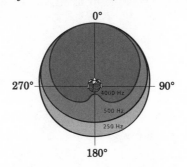

Figure courtesy of HGC
Engineering, Ltd.
Used with permission.

Figure 11-2: Directionality of the human voice

were to measure the sound pressure level of a person speaking, one would find that for the lower frequency vowels, such as /a/, there would not be much difference whether measured from in front or behind the person. By contrast, there would be a greater loss of power for the higher frequency sounds such as the consonant /s/.

When the wavelength of sound is large in comparison to the body of the radiating device, it tends to radiate uniformly in all directions. That's why you can put your subwoofer just about anywhere in the room, including behind a couch. Subwoofer wavelengths are longer than 10 feet, and they radiate in all directions. When the wavelength of sound is small in comparison to the body of the radiator it tends to beam like a flashlight or even a laser, for the very high frequency sounds. That is why you have to aim your bookshelf loudspeakers toward your favorite listening location!

That may also be why the bass instruments get less attention than the trumpets. The conductor can put them just about anywhere, but he has to be sure the trumpets are pointed in the right direction so that they communicate effectively with the hall and do not damage the hearing of nearby orchestra members.

2. Reflections

Hard, rigid, flat surfaces such as concrete, brick, stone, plaster, glass or water (like a quiet lake) are almost perfect reflectors or mirrors of sound. The general law of reflection (shown in Figure 11-3) is, "the angle of incidence equals the angle of reflection." After several reflections the sound becomes "lost" in the normal room noise. If all the room surfaces are very reflective, noise is amplified, because the sound reflects over and over again, persisting for a long time and increasing the acoustic energy present in the room. Think about the sound of children at a swimming pool, the din of a cocktail party in a hard surfaced reception area, or a rock band in a school gym.

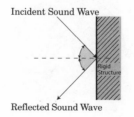

Incident Sound Wave

Rigid Structure

Reflected Sound Wave

Figure courtesy of HGC Engineering, Ltd. Used with permission.

Figure 11-3: The angle of incidence is equal to the angle of reflection

As a result of the law of reflection, convex surfaces tend to disperse sound over a larger area resulting in a more diffuse sound field that can be a desirable feature in music halls. Concave surfaces tend to concentrate or focus sound, a much less desirable effect (see Figure 11-4). Standing at the focal point of a dome or circular wall exemplifies this. All the sound is concentrated on you. Understanding this simple law of reflection allows architects to design spaces that are free from such unsettling effects, that we call acoustic defects.

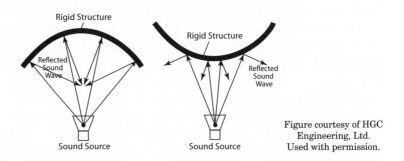

Figure 11-4: Reflections of sound rays from concave surfaces (on left) and convex surfaces (on right)

3. Source Location

The directivity and apparent strength of the source is also affected by its position in a room due to reflections from nearby large surfaces. The result is an increase in the sound pressure and the apparent loudness of the source even though the emitted sound power has not changed.

This is very possibly why some people suggest that loudspeakers sound better in the corner of the room. That is also why it's good to locate noisy equipment away from the walls, or to put sound absorbing material on the wall behind the equipment, thus decreasing the possibility of noise-induced hearing loss.

4. Standing Waves

When the distance between parallel room surfaces is equal to multiples of a half wavelength, those frequencies are accentuated. This is just a fancy way of saying that at certain points in the room, reflections off parallel surfaces, such as the ceiling and the floor, or two opposing walls, interact with each other and can create an undesirable increase in sound energy, much like ocean waves can interact to create a tidal wave. This is another way in which the room itself affects the distribution of sound pressure, and while this sounds technical, it essentially means that well-defined sounds will be undesirably enhanced in certain rooms. This is not generally a large problem in normal living rooms, but is of concern in critical listening rooms, such as recording studios, and can be a consideration in mechanical and equipment rooms where sound levels can become quite high at resonant frequencies if no absorption is present. If you have hearing loss, you'll want to discover which is the best room in your house for ideal hearing. For example, after dinner instead of lingering in the kitchen around highly reflective (hard) surfaces, the living room may be far more amenable as a good listening environment with all the soft absorbent surfaces.

5. Distance

In an outdoor environment or in a large room far from reflecting surfaces, a sound wave travels outward from its source in a spherical wave front. Consequently, its energy is spread over a continuously expanding surface. Since the area of a sphere is proportional to the square of its radius, the intensity of sound at any point is inversely proportional to the square of the distance from the source to that point. This becomes clearer when you realize that this is identical to how the light spreads out from a light bulb. For each doubling of the distance the intensity of the light beam decreases by one quarter. Eventually, like sound, the light is no longer noticed if the distance is great enough.

This is known as the *inverse square law* and it explains the decrease in loudness noticeable as you travel away from a source. When there are no reflecting surfaces, the reduction of sound pressure will be 6 dB each time the distance from the source is doubled.

As long as there are no significant reflecting surfaces, a sound (like a bothersome noise) that is twice as far away as another sound (like a voice) will be exactly 6 dB quieter. What this means is in the presence of noise, it will be easier for you to understand if you can shorten the distance between you and the speaker, and increase the distance from the noise. Thereby, distance can be very useful in controlling noise. Unfortunately, distance is always at a premium inside buildings and simply increasing the distance from the source to the receiver is not always an acceptable strategy. Also, inside workplaces there is generally a maximum distance from the source, called the *critical distance,* at which the sound level stops decreasing due to the effects of increased reflection off of the walls. This is called *reverberation.*

6. Reverberation

If all of the surfaces of a room were perfect reflectors of sound, all the sound energy in a room would bounce around forever and never die away. On the other hand, if all the surfaces of a room were perfect absorbers of sound, no reflections would occur and the decay of sound would be instantaneous. All rooms fall somewhere in between.

A useful measurement is called *reverberation time* and is defined as the length of time it takes sound to die away to a level of inaudibility after a sound source is turned off (see Figure 11-5). To quantify it more precisely, it's the time taken for sound to decay by 60 dB.

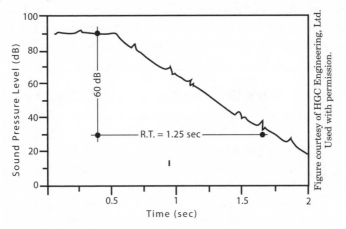

Figure 11-5: Reverberation Time (RT)

Reverberation occurs because sound travels at a finite speed of approximately 1,125 feet per second at room temperature. This is about one-third of a kilometer per second, or about 1/5 mile per second. If thunder is heard 5 seconds after the lightening in a storm, then the lightening was about a mile away. In a room whose walls, floor, and ceiling were about 33 feet apart, it would take sound approximately .03 seconds (or 30 milliseconds) to travel between them. So after 100 reflections, the initial sound will have lingered for 3 seconds. Add to that all the other sound which has occurred in the interim, and continues to linger, you can see that large reflective spaces can become very noisy due to the effects of reverberation—places to avoid with hearing loss.

This can have a very detrimental effect on speech and hearing. To hear speech, it requires a short reverberation time or the lingering sound energy will mask subsequent syllables and undermine intelligibility. Also, the amplification of noise due to reverberation can increase industrial sound levels in factories up to the harmful range. RTs that are too short may give the impression that the room is "dead" and those that are too long may cause the room to sound echoey.

We know that reverberation is stronger in large rooms, because it takes longer for the sound to travel between surfaces than in rooms with few absorptive surfaces. Specific equations can be used by acoustical engineers to determine what the reverberation time will be before a space is built, and to recommend corrective actions where required.

Preferred values of reverberation taken from several sources are presented in Table 11-1. Values are only approximate because of the large variation in spatial volume associated with facilities.

<u>Space/Performance</u>	<u>RT (seconds)</u>
Traditional Organ Music	2.5 – 5.0
Symphonic Repertoire	1.8 – 2.1
Chamber Music	1.6 – 1.8
Opera	1.3 – 1.6
Multipurpose Auditoriums	1.4 – 1.9
Live Theatre	0.9 – 1.4
Cinema Theatres	0.8 to 1.2
Classrooms	0.6 - 0.8
Lecture or Conference Rooms	0.6 - 1.1
Broadcast, Recording Studios	0.3 – 0.7

Table 11-1: Desired reverberation times (RT)

In spaces with excessive reverberation, sound levels don't decrease with distance from the source according to the well defined "inverse square law" and the entire workplace can become noisy and unpleasant. The critical distance is the location where the direct sound is equal to the reverberant sound, and it can be increased through the provision of acoustically absorptive materials to control reverberation.

If the walls and ceiling are treated with sound-absorbing material, the sound level in the reverberant field drops for the benefit of those located at some distance from the source. The sound levels near the source are not affected. One method of adding absorption to a manufacturing facility is through the use of hanging absorptive baffles. Another is perforated roof decking. If hearing loss in your workplace is preventing you from communicating effectively, reverberation issues should be considered.

Sound Absorption and the Noise Reduction Coefficient (NRC) Rating

We've talked about sound absorption and sound absorbing materials in several of the previous sections. The concept almost seems intuitive, but how does it work? Every time a sound wave is reflected, some of its energy is lost through absorption in the surface. The absorption is accomplished by changing sound energy into some other form, usually heat. Some surfaces absorb sound better than others. Soft porous materials like fabrics, people, fiberglass or mineral wool insulations, are examples of good acoustical absorbers. Being porous, they allow the sound waves to get inside the small pores and this introduces friction to the vibrating air molecules. For this reason, polystyrene (e.g., Styrofoam™) and other closed cell thermal insulations are not good acoustical absorbers because their cells are closed and the sound waves cannot directly enter them.

The amount of absorption provided by a particular surface material is generally frequency dependent and is rated by its sound absorption coefficients. These can vary between 0 and 1. If 50% of the energy is absorbed, the absorption coefficient is 0.5. Sound absorption coefficient values are generally listed at each of the standard octave band frequencies, 125, 250, 500 1000, 2000 and 4000 Hz. These are the primary frequencies audiologists assess when they test for hearing loss. These numbers correspond roughly to the octave below the middle of a piano keyboard (125 Hz) to the top note at the right side of the keyboard (4000 Hz). Sound absorption coefficients are determined through acoustical testing in an accredited acoustical laboratory, using established test methods contained in international and US standards (the American Society for Testing and Materials—ASTM)[1] If a material does not have published absorption coefficients, it should not be considered to be an acoustical treatment.

A shortcut is a single number rating of the absorption of a

material. This is the noise reduction coefficient (NRC) and is the average of the sound absorption coefficients at the 250, 500, 1000 and 2000 Hz, rounded to the nearest 0.05. This is often published on specification sheets for ceiling tile, carpet, roof decking, spray-on acoustic finishes, etc. and serves as a useful basis of comparison.

For sound to be absorbed, a good portion of the wavelength must actually be vibrating inside the material. That is why thin materials such as carpet only absorb high frequency (treble) sounds. The wavelength at 10,000 Hz (which is a little more than an octave above the top note of a piano keyboard) is approximately 1 inch, so carpet will be effective to absorb it, but carpet will have no effect on low frequency (long wavelength) sounds. The understanding of speech depends strongly on the clear intelligibility of speech consonants which are high frequency sounds. Using a thin absorber like carpet to control only high frequency sounds without controlling the low frequency vowels gives a space a "boomy" character in which speech is unbalanced and harder to understand. Progressive hearing loss due to normal aging or industrial noise exposure tends to initially affect high frequency hearing, complicating the situation. That's why carpet is not considered to be an acoustical material. Carpet manufacturers do not test and publish sound absorption coefficients for their products. Carpeting does a great job of cushioning footfall noise, such as the "clicking" of high heel shoes, so it's recommended for impact isolation, but not for acoustical absorption.

Thicker absorptive materials on the order of 2 inches thick are needed to control the lower frequencies as well and thereby control reverberation and activity noise in a more balanced way to enhance speech intelligibility. Very thick materials (up to a foot or more) are used in recording studios to control deep bass energy. Absorptive acoustical wall and ceiling treatments are available from suppliers in all major urban centers.

Acoustical ceiling tiles installed in a suspended T-Bar Ceiling System are another very popular way of absorbing sound and controlling noise within open office situations and classrooms. They form an integral part of a well designed open office area. The absorptive ceiling tiles reduce reflections over the partial height partitions between workstations. There are other types of acoustically absorptive finishes, furnishings and specialty products that aren't dealt with here. They're generally used in architecturally demanding applications outside the realm of noise control and the reader is referred to a good text on architectural acoustics.[2]

Sound Transmission between Rooms

One of the most annoying aspects of living in our modern society can be the sound created by our neighbors. Outdoor noise sources such as leaf blowers, pleasure craft, heavy traffic and motorcycles can enter buildings and interfere with work, sleep, concentration, and relaxation. The current trend toward lightweight or prefabricated building elements, saves space, cost, and construction time. However, this may come at the cost of annoyance or lack of privacy, because lightweight partitions transmit sound more effectively than the older, heavier construction. The use of drywall partitions between residential units, rather than concrete, is a good example. The term "partition" refers to any surface (wall, floor, door or window) that separates any two spaces horizontally or vertically.

When sound impacts a partition it is partially reflected and partially absorbed depending on the characteristics of the surface. The energy in the sound wave also causes the entire partition to vibrate. Remember that sound is a pressure wave, so it exerts an oscillating pressure (pushing force) on the partition which causes the vibration. The vibration may be small, but you can feel it if you place your fingers lightly on a wall if the volume and bass control of your stereo are turned up sufficiently loud. Don't do this without wearing hearing protection, or if your neighbors are home, or if you're worried about damaging your loudspeakers!

The sound transmission loss (TL) depends primarily on its mass and is simply the difference between measured sound levels on both sides of the partition in decibels (see Figure 11-6). When the partition vibrates it causes the air on its opposite side to be set into motion, creating sound in the adjacent space. The lighter the partition, the

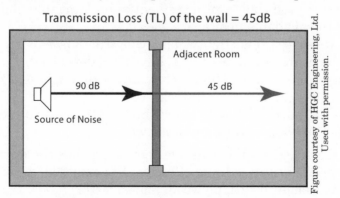

Figure 11-6: Demonstration of transmission loss (TL) through a partition

more it will move and the more sound will be radiated from its opposite surface.

Like most quantities in acoustics, the transmission loss depends on frequency, and in this case, transmission loss increases with frequency. Any partition is a much more effective insulator of sound at high frequencies than at low frequencies. Air gaps and leaks through adjacent building elements reduce the performance of actual construction below that of an ideal construction measured in the laboratory. Since hearing loss already poses hearing challenges, managing these barrier issues will improve communication and reduce stress for everyone.

Materials and Construction for Reducing Sound Transmission

When noisy spaces or areas (machine rooms, freeways, gymnasiums, party rooms) have to be situated close to quiet areas (bedrooms, libraries, conference rooms, executive offices) a potential acoustical conflict exists. Generally and as much as possible within the design program, architects try to position spaces within a building so that optimum acoustic performance is obtained without special construction. For example, corridors can be placed between mechanical rooms and living areas and less noise sensitive areas (kitchens, laundry rooms) can be placed between corridors and bedrooms. Where this is not possible, sound-insulating materials become more important.

The first thing one may think of is to use thicker walls, and that can certainly work, but it can be expensive. For example, a 6 inch thick concrete block wall has a Sound Transmission Class rating (STC 48), which does not meet most building code requirements. Doubling its thickness (mass) results in an improvement of 6 dB (STC 54), a good choice for a residential building, but the cost goes up and the available floor space goes down.

For these reasons, lightweight construction consisting of two leaves separated by an air space, have been developed. These can be designed to have a greater STC rating than single leaf partitions with less weight and overall thickness.

Two leaf partitions will achieve higher transmission losses than a single leaf wall of equal overall thickness if:

- Each leaf itself is massive enough and has the appropriate stiffness to be effective. For example, drywall or plaster board, plywood, and so forth.

- Maximum distance (air space) is provided between the leaves.
- Sound absorbing material (fiberglass or mineral wool batt insulation, for example) has been placed in the airspace.
- The connections points between the leaves are minimized and resilient connections are used.
- All leaks particularly around the perimeter have been carefully caulked and sealed. Even very small leaks can greatly undermine the STC rating.
- The partition does not contain components of lower transmission loss (light fixtures, electrical fixtures, windows, doors). The overall transmission loss of the partition is generally that of its weakest component.

Walls

There is a practical upper limit to the noise reduction possible from a wall in a typical structure. There are secondary transmission paths between rooms called *flanking transmission paths* (see Figure 11-7). When a partition has an STC of approximately 55–60, these flanking paths become important and dominate over the direct transmission path, so simply "beefing up" the wall will not improve the amount of noise reduction. Flanking paths are important consideration in the design of multi-residential buildings, schools and libraries.

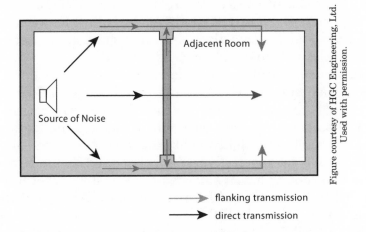

Figure courtesy of HGC Engineering, Ltd. Used with permission.

Figure 11-7: Transmission paths between rooms

The amount of noise reduction actually achieved in the open space will be different than the transmission loss through walls. This is because the actual noise reduction depends on the acoustic absorption present. The same amount of energy passing through a partition will create higher sound levels (and hence less noise reduction) in a very reverberant space than it would in a very absorbent room (a bedroom, for example). Engineering calculations to predict the noise reduction offered by a partition must therefore take the receiver room characteristics into account.

Floors and Ceilings

Special construction can be used to increase the sound insulation of floors and ceilings. A thick (8 inch) concrete slab is generally adequate for noise reduction in owner-occupied highrise condominiums but may be too massive for more lightweight residential structures. A concrete slab, on the other hand, offers poor impact isolation against footfall noise, such as the clicking of high heel shoes. To improve impact resistance a soft resilient surface such as carpet or rubber tile should be used.

Two methods are commonly in use to improve the transmission loss of concrete slab base building construction. The first is that a floating floor can be built above the existing structural slab. It can be made of wood or concrete, but concrete offers the best performance. This construction is often used between the mechanical rooms in highrise condominiums that are usually located immediately above the residential penthouse suites. All penetrations of the floating floor (ducts, pipes) are isolated to avoid short-circuiting between the structural floor and floating floor and all rigid contact between the floating floor and surrounding walls is avoided.

The second is that a suspended drywall ceiling is often used to achieve maximum noise reduction through a ceiling/floor assembly above a party room with suites above. The drywall ceiling is hung below the structural slab on resilient (spring) hangers and not affixed directly to it. Lightweight acoustic tile is a good absorber of sound, but it's not an effective noise barrier and should be avoided in a case like this, unless it's needed to control reverberation in the room below in which case both the drywall ceiling and the T-Bar ceiling can be used. The T-Bar ceiling should not be substituted for the drywall ceiling. The acoustic insulation is increased if sound-absorbing materials are used in the airspace. The number of suspension points should be kept to a minimum and the ceiling should not be penetrated by light fixtures or other objects. It should also be well caulked around the periphery with resilient caulking. Such a ceiling can improve the transmission loss of the entire partition by from 10 to 20 dB particularly at high frequencies. Keep in mind that it's the high frequencies in speech that give us intelligibility. Low frequencies give the power behind speech.

Windows

Windows are simply partitions, usually single or double, in the external facade of a building. All the comments made in previous sections about walls also apply to windows (improved transmission loss with thickness, and airspace). Generally, windows are designed to protect against traffic noise. Much research has been devoted to evaluating the effectiveness of various types of construction. A method developed by the National Research Council of Canada in 1980 is in common use for this purpose and to rate various window construction as to their acoustic effectiveness against traffic noise.[3] The analysis considers such factors as traffic sound levels, the window-to-floor area of the room in question and the placement of the facade in relation to the roadway. The sound insulation of windows increases with increased airspace and glazing thickness. The sound insulation of windows will also improve if absorption is included in the airspace, if unequal glass thicknesses are used and if the window units are nonoperable, but these are secondary effects.

Doors

To be acoustically effective, doors, that are usually the weak link in a partition, should be at least a solid core wood or insulated metal construction and well-sealed around the edges, including the threshold. Standard metal insulated exterior entry doors are well sealed, often with magnetic weatherstripping, and provide reasonable noise reduction at a budget price, but they're not provided with an STC rating. For high performance, STC rated doors are available from a number of specialty suppliers. These are designed and supplied with integral frames and with double sealing systems and are of a more massive construction. They're tested and guaranteed to provide a specific STC rating, and find application in recording studios, acoustical test facilities and high noise environments. Double door systems, such as those found between adjacent hotel suites are another option. Theaters, lecture halls, music practice rooms and recital halls often use sound locks (vestibules) with a door on each end to provide excellent isolation from the lobby or adjacent occupied space. Again with concern regarding hearing loss, if you're building a house or office space, it's good to keep these things in mind.

Control Measures for Noise Sources in Buildings

Indoor noise sources can broadly be separated into two categories: those produced by people (radio, TV, musical instruments, conversations) and those produced by mechanical equipment. Ways of reducing people-generated noise in residential buildings were discussed in previous sections of this chapter. This section addresses methods of controlling noise from mechanical equipment in buildings.

Noise from Plumbing Systems

Often when I'm traveling and need to stay in a hotel or motel, I don't need a wake-up call because I'm awakened by the sound of other guests using the shower. Does this sound familiar? Plumbing noise is often annoying. The radiation of noise and vibration from the pipes can be reduced by enclosing the pipes within drywall structures with insulation packed on the inside and by attaching them resiliently at their connection points. Special pipe wrappings can be used to reduce the amount of noise radiated directly from them. Pipes should never be allowed to touch or be rigidly attached to lightweight partitions (drywall, for example) or they'll cause the entire partition to radiate sound. The use of larger diameter pipes will result in reduced sound levels, but with the penalty of lower flow velocities.

Vibration Control

Vibration is becoming a greater concern in buildings with the increased use of thin and lightweight building materials, penthouse mounted mechanical rooms and long-span floors.

Vibration is noise and it can cause damage, be annoying, and interfere with work or sleep. Vibration isolation is generally achieved by placing springs between the vibrating equipment and the structural floor. These springs are called *vibration isolators* and take the form of coil springs (most effective) or rubber pads (least effective). There are vibration isolators available for small equipment like your furnace fan, to the largest roof-mounted chillers and cooling towers used to air condition highrise buildings and the standby power generators used for emergency purposes. When a machine is mounted on springs, the springs will compress due to the weight they have to support. The amount of compression is known as *static deflection*. Generally, more static deflection results in a greater amount of vibration isolation. It's very similar to the difference you feel between riding in an economy car and riding in a luxury vehicle with a "soft" suspension system.

Care must be taken however to avoid a situation known as *resonance*. Any mass on a spring will tend to vibrate almost spontaneously at a frequency known as the *resonant frequency* of the system. If the forcing frequency generated by the vibrating equipment is equal to this resonant frequency vibration, amplification can occur resulting in extremely high vibration levels and often structural damage. The more static deflection a system has, the lower the intensity of its resonant frequency. Needless to say, vibration isolation systems must be carefully designed to avoid resonance, yet provide sufficient static deflection to be effective.

Active Noise Control Systems

The control of noise by introducing "anti noise" or a second acoustical signal that is out of phase with the first, is known as *active noise control*. All of the noise control methods discussed previously were passive. They react to an acoustical signal in a manner that reduces its sound pressure, but requires no energy input to do so. Active noise control measures require a means of sampling the soundfield and a means of creating an out-of-phase cancellation signal.

The theoretical basis for active noise control has been known since the 1930s. Active noise control works best in very well-defined physical situations, such as sound generated by the detonations from an engine traveling down an exhaust pipe, or in very small spaces such as inside headphones. For these reasons it has found application in the automotive and aerospace industries, but there is currently little application in construction. Active noise control works by generating a sound that is 180° out of phase with the original sound. When the two are combined, sound cancellation occurs—thus silence.

It's like an ocean wave that intersects with a trough in the ocean, for a moment the wave has been cancelled out. Active noise control requires the use of loudspeakers whose output is designed to cancel the environmental noise.

Research is being actively conducted to use multiple loudspeakers to affect control over larger areas of space "zones of silence," and to use active vibration control for suspension systems and the control of radiating panels and other sound sources.

Commercial systems have recently become available for limited applications such as aircraft and automotive passenger compartments. The wide acceptance and development of low cost systems is being hindered by questions of universality and reliability. Active noise control has found application in noise control headsets for pilots but is only just starting to enter the general hearing protective device market served by low cost earplugs and muffs.

References

1. ASTM International. (2008) ASTM C423-08a-Statnd Test Method for Sound Absorption and Sound Absorption Coefficients by the Reverberation Room Method.
2. Egan DM. (2007) *Architectural Acoustics*. Florida: J. Ross Publishing
3. National Research Council of Canada. (1980) Acoustic Insulation Factor: A Rating for the Insulation of Buildings Against Outdoor Noise.

Glossary

acoustic trauma: rare condition where a single loud blast or explosion results in a permanent sensorineural (inner ear) hearing loss (also see *noise-induced hearing loss*)

Americans with Disabilities Act [1990] (ADA): specifically created to insure that "no individual shall be discriminated against on the basis of disability in the full and equal employment of the goods, services, facilities, privileges, advantages, or accommodations of any place or public accommodation"

ANSI: American National Standards Institute; body responsible for promulgation and maintenance of American national consensus standards

antiapoptotic: refers to the class of drugs that can prevent the process of apoptosis (see *apoptosis*)

antioxidant: a molecule capable of slowing or preventing oxidation which is a normal chemical reaction, but can produce free radicals that start chain reactions resulting in damage to cells (see *reactive oxygen species*)

apoptosis: one of two main methods by which cells die; the most common form of cell death from noise exposure; a passive disassembling of the cell where the components are gradually carried away; can also occur when the cell is separated from its surrounding cellular matrix (see *necrosis, antiapoptotic, reactive oxygen species*)

asymmetrical: not of equal proportion

ATF: Acoustical test fixture, known as acoustical or dummy head or acoustical manikins used for some hearing protector testing

attenuation: amount of reduction in noise level, such as that provided by use of a hearing protector, or other obstruction such as a wall

ATV: all-terrain vehicle, motorized quad vehicle that travels on low pressure tires, with a seat that is straddled by the operator, with handlebars for steering control

audiogram: graph to display a person's hearing thresholds with the test frequencies across the top and hearing loss (measured in dB HL) down the vertical axis; thresholds better than 25 dB HL are normal hearing

audiologist: one of a number of hearing healthcare professionals who have special graduate level training (either at the master's or doctorate level) in the assessment of hearing loss and the remediation of communication problems (also see *otolaryngologist*)

auditory nerve: the VIIIth cranial nerve that carries both balance and hearing information to the brain; all cranial nerves are denoted by their number in Roman numerals so VIII represents the 8th cranial nerve

balloon angioplasty and stent: technique of widening a narrowed or obstructed blood vessel by inflating a balloon catheter; frequently a small tube (stent) is then placed to keep the widened vessel open

basilar membrane: ribbon-like structure running the entire length of the cochlea; supports the organ of Corti; vibrations from the basilar membrane are transferred to hair cells in the Organ of Corti (also see *organ of Corti*)

bilateral: pertaining to both sides (or both ears)

binaural hearing: hearing using both ears; improves hearing something in a background of noise as well as helping to locate the source of a sound

brainstem: portion of the brain between spinal cord and cerebrum

cardiovascular disease (CVD): class of diseases involving the heart or blood vessels

characteristic frequency: auditory nerve fibers tuned very precisely to respond best to a certain frequency

cochlea: bony, snail-shaped auditory portion of the inner ear consisting of fluid-filled channels; contains approximately 15,000 nerve endings called hair cells; the primary sensory organ of hearing (see *inner ear*)

Code of Federal Regulations (CFR): annually revised accumulation of executive agency regulations published in the daily Federal Register combined with previously issued regulations still in effect; it is divided into 50 Titles with each representing a broad subject area and are the regulatory laws governing practice and procedure before federal administrative agencies

Cognitive Behavioral Therapy: attempts to solve emotional, behavioral or thought disorders through a psychotherapeutic approach

comparative negligence: negligence under law that is measured in the percentage of the plaintiff's/defendant's own negligence that may determine or offset certain awards or recovery to parties incurring an injury, damage, or death; courts will impute the percentage of negligence to each party in determining any ultimate award or damage

conductive hearing loss: any hearing loss due to a problem with the outer ear (e.g., wax) and/or middle ear (e.g., fluid); typically temporary; treatable medically or surgically by a physician, often an otologist (also see *sensorineural* and *otologist*)

congenital: existing as such from birth

contralateral: on the opposite side

contributory negligence: act or omission due to lack of ordinary care by the "damaged" party (plaintiff) that is legally required to conform to for his/her own protection; lack of exercised care may reduce or eliminate one's ability to obtain a cure for the defendant's negligence in the same matter

coronary bypass surgery: surgery in which a blocked coronary artery is bypassed utilizing a fresh, unclogged blood vessel taken from elsewhere (usually in the leg or chest of the patient)

critical distance: distance from a source in an enclosed space at which sound level of the direct sound is equal to the sound level of the reverberant sound (also thought of as the point at which the direct soundfield and the reverberant soundfield meet)

deaf: in North America, implies having no or limited useful hearing; often used as a term that is cultural rather than based on hearing loss; if the capital letter "D" is used it implies that a person-self-identifies with the "Deaf" community; in England and some parts of English-speaking Europe, this term refers to any hearing loss regardless of degree or etiology (also see *hard of hearing*)

decibel (dB): one-tenth of a bel; mathematical relationship between a measured sound pressure level and a reference sound pressure level; the reference is stated after the decibel, such as dB SPL

decibel A-weighted (dBA): a unit of noise measurement designed to approximate the response of the human ear to moderate sound pressure levels; also written as dB(A); the A-weighting adjustment is commonly used for noise measures because it approximates the human response to sound better than other commonly available measures; a special filter is used

decibel C-weighted (dBC): a unit of noise measurement designed to approximate the response of the human ear to high sound pressure levels; also written as dB(C), no filter is used on the sound level meter

decibel hearing level (dB HL, also written as dB HTL—hearing threshold level): level of hearing at a given frequency for an individual; the 0 dB HL reference is the average hearing of thousands of young adults recorded on an audiogram with no known hearing loss (see *audiogram*)

decibel sound pressure level (dB SPL): mathematical relationship between a measured sound pressure level and a reference sound pressure level of 0.0002 dynes/cm^2 (also see *sound pressure level*)

diplacusis: auditory injury characterized by abnormal pitch perception between the two ears; sufferer perceives a sound of a certain pitch in one ear is a little different from the pitch heard in the other ear, resulting in distorted sound perception

directivity: the three dimensional spatial directional characteristics of a sound source

dosimeter: (see *noise dosimeter*)

dysequilibrium: a sense that one's balance or equilibrium is not functioning properly

electroconvulsive shock therapy: procedure in which an electric current is passed through the brain of an anesthetized patient to produce controlled convulsions (seizures); predominantly used to treat patients with major depression unresponsive to other treatments and is rarely used today

Eustachian tube: narrow tube connecting middle ear to back of mouth; responsible for pressure equalization; dysfunction can result in middle ear infections or fluid

exchange rate: number of decibels that a noise level is increased when the exposure level has been doubled; a 3 dB exchange rate means that for each 3 dB increase in noise level, the exposure level has been doubled

external auditory meatus: canal of the ear that extends inwardly from the concha and terminates at a thin coned-shaped sheet of tissue—the eardrum—called the tympanic membrane (also see *outer ear*)

frequency: the number of vibrations (cycles per second) in a sound wave, also referred to as "Hz" (also see *pitch*)

habituation: process by which repeated and harmless stimulation leads to less and less perception and reaction, and seen in all organisms from very simple single-celled protozoa to humans

habituation-based therapy: any number of therapies directed at using habituation to minimize the effects of a troubling health concern such as tinnitus or hyperacusis

hair cells: sensory follicles of the cochlea housed within the organ of Corti; inner hair cells are primarily involved in transduction of sound to the brain; outer hair cells primarily receive impulses from the brain (see *organ of Corti*)

hard of hearing: refers to people with a hearing loss significant enough to cause communication difficulties and require some form of assistance/amplification (syn: hearing impaired)

Hearing Aid Compatibility Act: requires that all telephones manufactured after August 16, 1989 be compatible for use with the telecoils of hearing aids

Hearing Loss Prevention Act (1983): promulgated by the Occupational Safety and Health Administration (OSHA), this piece of legislation sets a maximum allowable noise dose to protect a large percentage of people; however, these regulations set only minimum safety standards, only apply to the occupational setting, and per OSHA admittedly do not protect a significant subset of the population

hearing protection device (HPD): collectively, devices that are worn on, over, or in the ears to attenuate sound in an effort to minimize its potential damaging effect on hearing

hearing threshold: the quietest sound audible 50% of the time when a person is undergoing a hearing test (see *audiogram*)

Hertz (Hz): a unit of frequency; the number of times that a wave passes a point each second; previously called cycles per second (CPS); the higher the value (e.g., 8000 Hz) the higher the frequency

hyperacusis: abnormally reduced tolerance to sound; a symptom where sound that is not especially loud, and not bothersome to other people, seems overwhelming, intense, or even painful

hysteria: generally refers to a personality disorder characterized by excessive emotions, dramatics, and attention-seeking behavior

Impact Isolation Class (IIC): a single number rating system that describes the ability of a floor/ceiling assembly to reduce the transmission of sound due to impacts such as footfalls or dropping objects

Individuals with Disabilities Education (IDEA): requires that children with disabilities be provided with a free and appropriate public education that includes special education and related services to meet the "unique" needs of children

inner ear: location of the cochlea, the sensory organ for hearing, and the vestibule, an organ responsible for balance (also see *cochlea*)

insomnia: sleep disturbance characterized by either difficulty falling asleep, awakening frequently during the night and staying awake, or waking too early; can be short-term (days to weeks) or chronic (months)

intensity: to increase in degree or force; relative to sound, the power transmitted through a medium

interaural difference: time or intensity differences between a signal reaching one ear before the other

ipsilateral: on the same side

ISO (International Standards Organization): international body responsible for promulgation and maintenance of international consensus standards

L_{eq} Equivalent noise level: the noise exposure level measured with a 3 dB exchange rate (see *exchange rate*)

localization: identification of the location of a sound source

L$_{OSHA}$: equivalent noise level measured with a 5 dB exchange rate

loudness: perception or impression of the strength of a sound without reference to any physical measuring tool such as a sound level meter (see *intensity,* and *sound pressure level*)

masker: sound source that interferes with the perception of another sound

masking: interfering with the perception of one sound by another; the level of interference that one sound can affect on another

middle ear: portion of ear between the eardrum and inner ear; air space comprised of three tiny bones (malleus, incus and stapes)

misophonia: aversion to sound (see *hyperacusis*)

MP3 player: digital audio device with primary function of storing, organizing and playing <u>audio files</u>, some with image-viewing and/or video-playing support

NASCAR: National Association for Stock Car Auto Racing, a family-owned and operated business that operates many <u>auto racing</u> sports events

National Institutes of Occupational Safety and Health (NIOSH): a federal US agency part of the Centers for Disease Control (CDC) within the US Department of Health and Human Services (DHHS); focus is neither regulatory nor issues safety and health standards, but conducts research and develops safety and health regulations with a goal of preventing work-related illnesses and injury, including those potentially due to hearing and hearing loss considerations (see *Occupational Safety and Health Act*)

necrosis: form of cell death where the cell swells and explodes allowing its internal contents and cytoplasm to spread beyond its boundaries and cause toxicity in the neighborhood of other cells (see *apoptosis, reactive oxygen species*)

negligence: failure to use such care as a reasonably prudent and careful person would use; these actions may range from intentional actions to unintended omissions, but fall below the accepted level of conduct or action; in the healthcare arena, usually involves the failure to act or perform to an accepted and recognized standard of care

nephrotoxicity: property of a natural or artificial substance that damages the kidney

neurosis: mental disorder that triggers feelings of distress and anxiety, but does not include delusions or hallucinations (see *psychosis*)

neurotoxicity: property of a natural or artificial substance that damages the nervous system

noise: sound with no particular information; in contrast to a signal such as speech or music, noise has random phase

Noise Control Act (1972): states that Americans are not to be subjected to noises that jeopardize health and well-being

noise dose: combination of sound level over time that describes sound exposure; expressed as a percentage of maximum allowable exposure where 100% constitutes maximum allowed

noise dosimeter: specialized sound level meter that measures noise exposure (in dBA) over time and integrates the total exposures so that the result is representative of the risk; worn by a person concerned about the possibility of losing hearing based on the level of a specific noise exposure

noise-induced hearing loss (NIHL): most common preventable source of sensorineural hearing loss caused by long-term exposure to sound in excess of 85 dBA; cumulative throughout one's lifetime characterized by decreased hearing sensitivity, tinnitus, hyperacusis, and/or diplacusis (see *acoustic trauma*)

Noise Reduction Coefficient (NRC): single number rating that describes the ability of an acoustical wall or ceiling treatment material to reduce the noise in the reverberant field of a room through absorption; the average of the 250 Hz, 500 Hz, 1000 Hz, and 2000 Hz absorption coefficients rounded (obtained through laboratory testing and rounded to the nearest 0.05)

Occupational Safety and Health Act (1970): designed to reduce incidences of personal injuries, illnesses, and deaths within the occupational setting; the Occupational Safety and Health Administration (OSHA) is a federal agency in the United States created by this act

Occupational Safety and Health Administration (OSHA): federal agency in the US created by the Occupational Safety and Health Act, developed to enact occupational safety and health standards and regulations, conduct investigations and inspections to determine compliance with established safety and health regulations, and issue citations and penalties for noncompliance (see *Occupational Safety and Health Act—1970*)

Office of Noise Abatement and Control (ONAC): American federal program established in the Environmental Protection Agency (EPA) to monitor the Noise Control Act (1972); federal funding removed in 1980

organ of Corti: complex structure within the cochlea that sits on the basilar membrane and contains hair cells and other structures necessary to transmit sounds to the auditory or hearing nerve; two types of hair cells are the inner hair cells and the outer hair cells, named because of their locations within this structure (see *basilar membrane* and *scala media*)

otoacoustic emissions (OAE): emissions that emanate from the auditory system and can be measured with sophisticated microphones situated in the outer ear canal; their discovery in the late 1970s resulted in development of clinical audiology tests

otolaryngologist (ear, nose, throat): medical doctor with residency specialty training in the medical and surgical problems of the ear, nose, throat, head and neck (syn. ENT doctor, ear doctor)

ototoxicant: man-made substance able to damage an exposed organism, or part of it

ototoxicity: property of a substance that causes damage to the ear

ototraumatic: broader term than the term ototoxic; used in hearing loss prevention, refers to any agent (e.g., noise, drugs or industrial chemicals) that has the potential to cause permanent hearing loss subsequent to acute or prolonged exposure

outer ear: most external area from the cartilaginous portion outside of ear through to the eardrum (also see *external auditory meatus)*

permanent threshold shift (PTS): permanent and irreversible hearing loss resulting from excessive exposure to noise (see *sensorineural hearing loss,* and *temporary threshold shift*)

personal listening device (PLD): a portable device that plays cassette tapes, compact discs, MP3 file format music or other audio content, and is used via headphones in the form of on-the-ear headphones, earbud earphones, etc.

pesticide: any chemical used to kill insects or weeds

phonophobia: fear of loud sounds (see *hyperacusis*)

pitch: psychological counterpart to frequency, essentially means the same thing (also see *frequency*)

polysomnagram: an overnight sleep study usually done at a sleep disorders center

potentiation: action in which a substance or physical agent at a concentration or dose that does not itself have an adverse effect, enhances the harm done by another substance or physical agent

presbycusis: most common sensorineural hearing loss associated with aging (see *sensorineural hearing loss*)

products liability: legal liability of manufacturers and sellers to compensate buyers, users, and even bystanders for damages or injuries suffered because of defects in goods purchased

propagation: phenomenon by which the motion of the original vibrating surface "travels" as a wave in all directions provided there is a medium

psychosis: mental disorder characterized by a loss of contact with reality and, in which people often experience hallucinations or delusions (see *neurosis*)

pulsatile tinnitus: perception of abnormal pulsing sounds (resembling one's heartbeat) in the ears or head; usually caused by blood flow disturbance, a blood vessel abnormality, or more uncommonly a vascular tumor (see *tinnitus*)

pure tone: sound wave having only one frequency of vibration

pure tone audiometry: measurement of hearing sensitivity thresholds to pure-tone presentations by air or bone conduction (see *audiogram*)

quiet enjoyment: covenant in conveyances promising a tenant or owner of a premises that they may use it in peace and without disturbance, but when the covenant is violated, there is a mechanism to seek relief

reactive oxygen species (ROS): free radicals that are caused during normal cellular oxidation and results in damage to certain structures such as the hair cells in the inner ear; generation of free radicals has been associated with cellular injury in different organ systems; considered a basic mechanism of toxicity (see *antioxidant*)

REAT: (real ear attenuation at threshold), a procedure for estimating hearing protection attenuation by providing a hearing threshold test with and without hearing protectors in place and comparing the results

recruitment: when a slight increase in the intensity of sound seems disproportionately greater

Rehabilitation Act of 1973: requires that programs receiving federal funds be used by people with disabilities; thus the federal government cannot operate in a discriminatory manner

Reissner's membrane: separates the scala vestibule from the scala media

reverberation: prolongation of sound by multiple reflections after the original sound has been removed

scala media: middle portion of the cochlea that houses the endolymph-filled organ of Corti; bordered on the bottom by the basilar membrane and the top by Reissner's membrane (see *organ of Corti*)

scala tympani: lower portion of the cochlea filled with perilymph fluid; bordered on the top by the basilar membrane

scala vestibuli: top portion of the cochlea filled with perilymph fluid; bordered on the bottom by Reissner's membrane; the stapes footplate vibrates in and out of the oval window which is the entrance to the scala vestibuli

sensorineural hearing loss: diminished hearing sensitivity due to injury or medical condition affecting the inner ear or the auditory nerve that connects the inner ear to the brain (i.e., the cochlea and the VIIIth nerve); almost always a permanent, non-medically treatable disorder (see *permanent threshold shift,* and *conductive hearing loss*)

signal: sound that we are trying to hear; typically has non-random phase

signal to noise ratio (SNR or S/N): calculated as the difference (in decibels) between the signal level and the noise level; positive SNR (e.g., +5 dB SNR) indicates the signal is more intense than the noise; can also be a negative ratio (e.g., -5 dB SNR)

simultaneous masking: interference with the perception of a sound by another sound that is present at the same time

sound: particle vibrations in an elastic medium

sound absorption coefficient: set of dimensionless values from 0 to 1 that describe the ability of a material to absorb sound at each of the standard octave band frequencies

sound generator: in its application to tinnitus treatment, generates a (digital) recording of soothing sounds that might include rain, ocean waves, or forest sounds, to be played quietly at night to reduce the awareness of tinnitus; can also be worn in form of a "hearing aid" during waking hours to help minimize the tinnitus (see *tinnitus masker,* and *habituation*)

sound level meter (SLM): device that measures sound levels in decibels

sound power: acoustic power output of a sound source measured in watts

sound power level: a measurement of sound watts level (SWL), also described as level of watts (L_W) that quantifies sound power measured on a logarithmic decibel scale (dB); equal to 10 times the logarithm to the base 10 of the ratio of the sound power of the source to a reference sound power which is normally taken to be 10^{-12} watt = 0 dB SWL in air

sound pressure: local pressure deviation from the ambient (average) pressure caused by a sound wave measured using a microphone

sound pressure level (SPL or Lp): quantity of sound pressure measured on a logarithmic decibel scale relative to the reference of 0.0002 dynes/cm^2 (also see *decibel sound pressure level*)

sound transmission class: single number rating system that describes the ability of a building partition (wall, floor, etc.) to reduce the transmission of airborne sound

standards: application of some measure, principle, practice, or other approach by which things of the same class are compared in order to determine their quality, quantity, value, etc.

standing wave (also known as a stationary wave): a <u>wave</u> that remains in a constant position as a result of <u>interference</u> between two waves traveling in opposite directions; most typically occurs due to reflections in rooms with large parallel reflective surfaces when distance between those surfaces is equal to multiples of a half wavelength; consequence of standing waves in normal size rooms is that some low frequency (bass) notes sound louder in specific places

statute: formal written enactment of a legislative body at the federal, state, or local level

sterocilia: rigid hairlike projections rooted in the apical end of the inner and outer hair cells

stria vascularis: network of capillaries that form the outer wall within the scala media

strict liability: liability without fault; covers a wide variety of concepts including Workers' Compensation, Product Liability, and injury from activities known to be "ultra hazardous" by their nature (e.g., blasting)

subject matter experts (SMEs): consider new scientific developments in the field, new technologies, the applicability of the standard and their technical aspects, and how the standard has been used by end-users

superior olivary complex: collection of auditory nerve fibers relaying information from the cochlea to the brain

synergism: interaction in which the combined biological effect of two or more substances is greater than expected on the basis of the simple sum of the toxicity of each of the individual hazards

synergistic effects: biological effects following combined exposure to two or more substances that is greater than the simple sum of the effects that occur following exposure to the substances separately

tectorial membrane: cellular, gelatinous-like structure in contact with the outer hair cells, but not the inner connected on the inner side of the organ of Corti

Telecommunications Act of 1996: requires television programming including broadcast, cable and satellite to follow a specific schedule (over a period of eight years and beginning in 1998) for providing captioning

Teletypewriter (TTY) or Telecommunications Device for the Deaf (TDD): an electronic device for text communication transmitted over a telephone line that a hard of hearing person may use as a substitute for a telephone; can be about the size of a laptop computer and allows coupling to a telephone; often used in conjunction with a telephone relay service that makes it possible to successfully call regular telephone users

Television Decoder Circuitry Act: required all television sets with screens 13 inches or larger, manufactured or imported into the United States after July 1, 1993, to be capable of displaying closed-captioned television transmissions

temporal masking: masking produced by a noise that occurs either just before or just after the signal occurs

temporary threshold shift (TTS): reversible hearing loss from a single exposure to loud noise; usually of brief duration, lasting several hours to days, and completely resolves (see *permanent threshold shift*)

threshold: quietest sound audible 50% of the time (see *hearing threshold,* and *REAT*)

tinnitus: (pronounced tih-NEYE'-tuhs or TIHN'-ih-tuhs, derived from the Latin verb *tinnire*—to ring), sensation of ringing, buzzing, whooshing or other sound in the ears or head without an external stimulus; a symptom that is the conscious expression of a sound that originates in an involuntary manner in the head of its owner, or may appear to him to do so; may take on many forms ranging from tone-like sound to any noise such as static or wind; may be constant or intermittent (see *pulsatile tinnitus*)

tinnitus maskers: older approach to minimizing the effects of tinnitus by using higher volume of sound to completely cover the tinnitus (see *sound generators*)

tonotopic organization: spatial arrangement along the organ of Corti according to tonal frequency; also pertains to structures within the peripheral and central auditory nervous system

torts: Latin word meaning "twisted wrong;" a private or civil remedy for a wrong or injury resulting form a violation of a duty through actions under operation of law

toxicant: man-made substance that is able to damage an exposed organism, or part of it

toxicity: property of a substance to cause damage to a living organism; can refer to the effect on a whole organism, such as an animal, bacterium, or plant, as well as the effect on a substructure of an organism

toxin: substance that is able to damage an exposed organism, produced by living cells or organisms

unilateral: pertaining to one side only (or one ear)

upward spread of masking: masking of high frequency sounds by low frequency maskers; amount of upward spread of masking increases with higher intensity maskers

vertigo: (from the Latin verb *to turn*), hallucination of motion when no motion is occurring

vestibular: having to do with the body's system of maintaining balance; generally used in reference to that portion of the balance system related to the inner ear

word recognition testing: formerly referred to as "speech discrimination testing;" one of a number of tests performed by an audiologist during a hearing assessment; a number of well-defined words spoken to a patient who responds with what they hear; percentage correct is the word recognition score

Index

A

absolute zero, 12
absorptive materials, 170-80
acetylsalicylic acid, 92
acoustic neuroma, 118
acoustic reflexes, 91
acoustic trauma, 9, 10, 51, 56, 58, 66, 115
Acoustical Society of America, 155
acoustical test fixtures, 157
Acoustics and Noise Control, 155
active noise control, 180
Age Discrim in Employ Act, 133
Alzheimer's disease, 98, 123
Amer Conf of Gov'tl Indust Hygienists, 100
Amer Nat'l Standards Inst, 40, 154-57, 159-61
Amer Soc for Testing and Materials, 59, 171
Amer Sp-Lang-Hear Assn, 40-41
Amer Tinnitus Assn, 113
Americans with Dis Act, 133-36, 138
  Title I, 134
  Title II, 135
  Title III, 135
  Title IV, 135
anatomy (physiology), 16-31
antibiotics,
  aminoglycoside, 92-93, 117
  streptomycin, 92
antidepressants (see *tinnitus-*)
anti-inflammatories,
  nonsteroidal, 117
Anti-Kickback Statutes, 142
anti-malaria (drugs), 93
anti-noise, 33-34
antioxidants, 10, 98-99, 118
  glutathione, 98
anvil (see *incus*)
architects, 45
architectural strategies (also see *sound pressure levels*), 163-180
applying, 164
  sound power and, 164-65
  sound pressure and, 164-65
asphyxiants (see *chemicals, industrial*)
aspirin, 117, 121
assistive listening devices, 143
audiogram, 4-6, 15, 109
  frequencies on, 4-5
  ototoxic configuration on, 93
audiologist, 56, 64, 67-69, 71, 93, 101, 109, 171
  defined, 3
audiological testing, 6, 118
audiometers, 7
audiometry,
  defined, 3, 94
auditory nerve, 16, 25, 28-29
aural rehabilitation, 10, 118
autoimmune disorders, 118
A-weighted dBA (see *decibel scale*)

B

background noise (see *noise*)
balance, 28, 118
basilar membrane, 21-23, 26-27
binaural hearing (see *hearing*)
binaural summation (see *hearing*)
British Tinnitus Assn, 113
Brownian motion, 12

C

Canadian Standards Assn, 154
cardiovascular disease, 117-18
CAT scan, 118
cease and desist orders, 142
ceilings, acoustical, 38-39, 167, 169, 171-72, 176-77
Center for Disease Control, 115, 133
central auditory pathway, 17, 29-30
Central Michigan Univ, 56
cerebrospinal fluid, 22
cerumen, impaction of, 5
characteristic frequency, 29
chemicals (see *industrial-*)

chemotherapeutics, 93, 117
chemicals, industrial, 92-102
  acrylonitrile, 95, 97
  asphyxiants, 93
  carbon disulphide, 96, 101
  carbon monoxide, 97-99, 117
  chlorobenzene, 96
  degreasers, 94
  ethylbenzene, 96
  fuels, 94, 101
  hydrogen cyanide, 95, 97, 99,
    101, 117
  iminodipropionitrile, 97
  insecticides, 95
  lead, 97, 100-101
  manganese, 100
  mercury, 97, 101
  metals, 93, 98
  nephrotoxicity from, 98
  neurotoxicity from, 98
  n-butyl alcohol, 100
  n-heptane, 96
  n-hexane, 96, 101
  organic tin, 101
  organotins, 97
  paint, 94
  paint thinners, 94
  pesticides, 93, 97-98, 101
  poisons, 95
  polychlorinated biphenyls, 93, 97
  polyurethanes, 94
  protection from, 100-101
  solvents, 93-94, 98
  styrene, 96, 101
  toluene, 96, 100-101
  toxicants, 93
  trichloroethylene, 96
  trimethyltins, 97
  xylenes, 96, 101
cisplatin, 93
Civil Rights Act, 133
claims (see *tort laws*)
cochlea (also see *inner ear*), 17, 21-
  28
  hair cells in, 22-23, 51
    bundles of, 24
    function of, 25, 26-28
    number of, 25
    sound hitting, 35, 115
  high pitch areas of, 17, 80
  inner hair cells of, 21, 23-24, 28
    number of, 25
    shape of, 24
  low pitch areas, 80
  outer hair cells of, 21, 23-24
    number of, 25
    shape of, 24
cochlear nuclei, 30
cognitive function, 11
communication, 3, 174
  improving, 87-90
concha, 17-18
cochlear nerves, 18
consonants (also see *frequency*),
  high frequency, 4, 18, 28, 116,
    166, 172
  low frequency, 4, 18
  sibilant, 18
Council on the Environment of NY,
  36
cranial nerve, 28
cuticular plate, 24

D

dB exchange rate, 9-11, 13-14
dBA (see *decibel scale*)
decibels, 6, 8
decibel scale, 7, 51, 57
  A-weighted, 51, 159, 165, 184
  C-weighted, 159, 184
Deiter cells, 23
Dept of Environ Protect of NYC, 41
diabetes, 117
diplacusis, 52
diuretics, 93
  loop, 117
dizziness (also see *noise, exposure
  to*) 92
doors, 177-78
dosimeters, 14, 59, 67, 161

E

ear,
 discharge in, 117
 external (see *outer*)
 fullness in, 117
 inner, 17-18
 middle, 5-6, 16-22
  negative pressure in, 19
 outer, 17-19
 pain in, 117
earbuds, 62, 64, 83, 145
eardrum, 5-6, 17, 19
 perforation of, 5
 rupture of, 19
 sound hitting the, 12, 35
ear infections, 5-6
 altitude changes and, 5
earmuffs, 68-69, 118, 157-58, 180
earphones (also see *noise: head
  phones*), 64, 70-71, 145
 sound isolating- 71
earplugs, 56, 68-70, 118, 180
 Musicians Earplugs™, 69
earwax (see *cerumen*)
educational development, 11
eighth nerve, 25, 28, 35
endolymph fluid, 22-23, 25, 93
Environmental Protection Agency,
  14, 33, 37, 42, 44, 52, 131-32
European Environmental Agency, 15
European Union, 153
Eustachean tube, 5, 19
explosions, 11
exposure (see *noise*)

F

False Claims Act, 142
Fed Aviation Admin (FAA), 34-35,
  42, 43
Fed Interagency Comm on Aviation
  Noise, 40
filter (see *decibel scale*)
fireworks, 11
flavonoids, 99
floors, 176-77

G

Food and Drug Admin, 11
free radicals, 10, 98-99, 115
frequency, defining, 3
 high, 4, 7, 27-30
 low, 4, 7, 27-30, 71
 mid, 27

G

gender, 117
genetic factors, 117
Going Green, 140
green efforts, 141
Green High-Perf Schl Facilties Act,
  41
Guidelines for Comm Noise, 139
gunfire, 10

H

hair cells (see *cochlea*)
hair dryers, 13
hammer (see *malleus*)
headphones (also see *noise; noise
  cancellation*), 70-71, 83-84, 103
head trauma, 117
Hear Education and Awareness for
  Rockers, 65
hearing, 1-15, 28
 basics of, 1-15
 binaural (summation), 83-84, 86
 measurement of, 1-15, 67
Hear Aid Compatability Act, 135
hearing aids, 10, 61, 118
hearing conservation programs, 45,
  50
hearing level,
 defined, 6-7
hearing loss, 1-15, 32, 45, 49-74,
  94, 114-28
 acoustic trauma type (also see
  acoustic trauma), 115
 asymmetrical, 60
 chronic noise-induced, 115
 children with, 36-41, 50, 52-54,
  60-61, 75
 conductive type of, 5-6

basics of, 1-15
high frequency, 53,
measurement of, 1-15
occupational, 67
recreational noise and, 49-74
sensorineural type of, 5-6, 11
treatment for, 118-19
types of noise-induced, 115
hearing protection (also see *ear-muffs; earplugs*), 10, 57, 68, 89, 150-162
hearing protectors (also see *noise: standards*), 150-162
hearing threshold level (see *hearing level*)
heart issues,
fetal, 11
Heathrow Airport, 40, 43
heliocotrema, 22
Hertz (Hz), 3
high blood pressure (see *noise*)
high frequencies (see *frequency*)
hearing protection for, 69
inner hair cells for, 21, 23-24, 28
need for, 116
hyperacusis (see *tinnitus*),
Hyperacusis Network, 104, 111, 113
hyperlipoproteinemia, 117
hypertension (see *noise, high blood pressure*)
hypothyroidism, 118

I

incus, 20-21
Individ with Disabil Ed, 135-36
industrial chemicals (see *chemicals*)
industrial noise (see *noise, indust.*)
inner ear (also see *cochlea*), 5-6, 10, 22, 91
insomnia (see *tinnitus*)
interaural time, 84-85
Int'l Standards Organ, 154-55, 157-59, 161-62
inverse square law, 88, 168, 170
iPods® (see *noise*)

L

lawn mowers, 13
law(s) (also see *legal*),
Dictionary of (Black's), 130
healthcare and the, 131
hierarchy of, 130-31
noncompliance with, 142
Quiet Enjoyment, 147
whistleblower, 142
legal (also see *laws*)
-enactments, 131
-implications, 141-47
L-N-acetyl-L-cystine, 10
Lindsay, Mayor John, 39
linear, 7
Listen Up!, 53-54, 61, 72
litigation, 66
Lombard effect, 88
low frequency (see *frequency*)
lowest observed adverse effect level, 94
Lowey, Nita, 34

M

macular degeneration, 99
Magnetic Resonance Imaging, 109, 118
malleus, 20-21
masking, 81-102
backward, 81
duration of, 81
forward, 80-81
hearing speech during, 81-102
high intensity, 76-80, 82-83, 86
loudness of, 82-83
low intensity, 76-77, 79-80
simultaneous, 81
temporal, 80-81
medical consequences of noise, 114-28
metabolism, 10
middle ear (see *ear*)
military exposure (see *noise*)
Military Whistleblower Act, 142
MP3 (see *noise*)

music (see *noise*)
frequencies of, 18
Musicians' Clinics of Canada, 72
musicians hearing program, 72

N

NASCAR (see *noise*)
Nat'l Environ Policy Act, 131
Nat'l Hear Conserv Assn, 72
Nat'l Inst for Deafness and other Comm Dis, 52
Nat'l Inst of Health, 50, 52
Nat'l Inst of Occup Saf and Health, 133
Nat'l Research Council of Canada, 177
negligence (see *tort laws*)
neoplasms, 117
neurological impulses, 23
neurotoxicity, 92-102
NJ Citizens for Abatement of Aircraft Noise, 34
NoBoomers, 44
No Fear Act, 142
noise,
agricultural, 136
air compressor, 57
air conditioner, 76
aircraft, 32, 36-40, 136, 143
airports and, 36, 138
annoying, 35
arcade game, 117
ATV, 58
auto alarm, 41
background, 5, 28, 64-65, 67, 75-102, 116
band, 54
band saw, 57
bar, 45
bench top planer, 57
blasting, 143
blenders, 13
boom car (also see *car stereo*), 32, 42,
bothersome, 35

brad nailer, 57
car stereo, 54-55, 82
CD player, 62
cell phone (see *telephone*)
chain saw, 57-58
chemicals and, 92-102
children and (see *noise, expos.*)
circular saw, 57-58
city, 138
cocktail party (see *party*)
concert, 54, 65
continuous, 51
conversational, 178
crowd, 65
dance club, 65-66
discomfort of, 19
disturbing, 35-36
defining, 2
drill press, 57
dust collector, 57
equipment, 178
explosive, 115
factory (see *industrial*)
firearm, 54-57, 115, 117-18
firecracker, 60, 145
four-wheeling, 50
gunfire (see *firearm*)
hair dryer, 58
hearing in, 75-102
highways and, 36
household, 13
hunting (see *firearm*)
impact, 98
improving communication in, 87-91
impulsive, 51
industrial, 8-9, 33, 44-45, 50, 138, 143
intrusive, 35
iPod,® 61-62, 145
jet (see *airplane*)
jet ski, 54-55, 58
jointer, 57
kitchen appliance, 58
laws and (see *laws*)

lawnmower, 54-55, 88
leaf blower, 54-55, 88, 173
legislating, 50
loudspeaker, 65
low frequency, 43
machinery, 33, 118
military, 3, 50
miter saw, 57
monster truck, 54, 58
motorcycle, 42-43, 54-55, 58, 173
motor sports, 58, 117
MP3, 3-4, 13, 67, 70, 119, 137,
    145
music as, 16, 38, 60-66, 76, 82-
    83, 85, 118, 136-37
musical instrument, 58, 60-65,
    178
narrowband, 77
NASCAR races and, 50, 58, 65-
    66
nightclub (see *party*)
party, 86, 94, 136
personal listening system, 61,
    119
plumbing, 178
power tool, 117
prevention of, 67-71
raceways and, 36
radio, 82, 88, 178
random phase, 3
restaurant, 45, 86, 94
rifle (also see *firearm*), 56
router, 57
sander, 57
shooting, 50, 68
shop vac, 57
signal to (see *sig. to noise ratio*)
snow blower, 88
snowmobiling, 50, 54-55
social levels of (see *party*)
solving, 39, 140-41
sound and, 34-35
spindle sander, 57
sporting event, 58-59
subway, 39

susceptibility to, 51, 59
table saw, 57
telephone, 137
television, 33, 38, 76, 178
toys that emit, 59-60
tractor, 54
traffic, 32, 36, 39, 50, 76, 86,
    136, 173
train, 33, 38-39, 136
train horn, 38
transportation, 33, 136
truck, 33
vacuum cleaner, 58
vibration (also see *vibrations*),
    178
voices as, 76
women around, 55
woodworking, 50, 57-58, 60
exposure to,
    aggression from, 42-43
    anger from, 42-43
    annoyance with, 173
    anxiety from, 44
    birth defects and, 137
    blood pressure and (see *high*-)
    bodily reactions from, 32-48
    boilermaker's deafness from,
        49
    buildings with, 178
    cardiovascular changes from,
        36, 137-38
    children and, 36-41, 50, 138
    circulatory changes from, 36
    cognitive impairment during,
        40, 137-38
    colitis from, 43
    communication during, 45
    concentration during, 173
    control of, 179-80
    crimes resulting from, 44
    criteria for, 8-9
    dangerous, 14, 19, 32-48
    disruption from, 32
    distress from (see *stress*)
    dizziness from, 137-38

duration of, 8-11
excessive hormones from, 36
fatigue and, 137
headaches from, 44, 137
headphone, 50, 55, 60-61, 64
heartburn from, 43
heart rate changes from, 36
helplessness from, 42-43
high blood pressure from,
    36-37, 40, 137
hopelessness from, 36
hypersensitivity during, 40
illnesses from, 36-37
immune system changes
    from, 137-38
indigestion from, 43
infants and, 37
irritability from, 44, 137
law enforcement and, 44
learning disabilities from, 137
long-term, 8-11
lower levels of, 11, 13
medical consequences of, 114-
    28
medical considerations of,
    136-39
medical evaluation for, 117-
    18
mental stress from, 42-43
morale and (see *poor-*)
motivational impairment dur-
    ing, 40
muscular pain from, 43
musculoskeletal disorders
    from, 45
neighborhoods and, 36-37
nervousness from, 42-43
non-auditory effects from,
    32, 34, 40, 50
occupational, 3, 6, 8-9, 50,
    52, 67, 99, 101, 132, 136,
    141, 150-162
offices during, 45
out-of-phase cancellation for,
    179

pain from, 137
partitions to prevent, 173-74
physical damage caused by,
    32-48
pleasures impacted by, 38
poor classroom performance
    from, 40
poor incidental memory
    from, 40
poor intentional memory
    from, 40
poor morale and, 45
poor performance during, 45,
    137
postural adjustments from,
    45
productivity and (see *poor-*)
psychophysical complaints
    from, 138
quality of life and, 37-38
reading and, 39
recreational, 3,6, 33, 49-74,
    117
    risks of, 52-55
regulating, 9, 11, 13, 49-50,
    100
relaxation issues with, 173
    safe, 9
sleep deprivation from, 32,
    36, 44, 137-38, 173
speech perception during, 85
stressful reactions from, 11,
    35-36, 42-44, 94, 98, 105,
    107-110, 124-27, 137-38,
    143-44, 174
sound cancellation (see *out-
    of-phase*)
sound level of, 8-9, 13
standards for, 50, 139-41,
    150-62
    by country, 149
    construction safety, 155
    defining, 151
    development of, 151-53
    hearing protection, 155-62

int'l, 153
measurement, 156-62
national, 153
organization of, 154-55
subject matter experts
on, 152-54
use of, 153-54
who develops, 154-55
telephone interference from,
38
television interference from,
38
tension from, 44
ulcers from, 43, 137-38
upset from, 44
urinary epinephrine levels
and, 45
vasoconstriction from, 137
vertigo from, 137
vibro-acoustic disease from,
43
walls to reduce, 175-76
warning devices during, 45
well-being jeopardized from,
37, 45
workplace, 44
young adults', 7
Noise: A Health Problem, 36, 41
Noise and Children, 37
Noise and Health, 43
noise cancellation, 71
noise codes, 33
noise complaints, 33
noise control, 67
Noise Control Act of 1972, 33, 133
noise dose, 51, 59, 66
noise dosimeter (see *dosimeters*)
Noise Exposure Standard, 155
Noise-Off, 34, 44
Noise Pollution Clearinghouse, 34
Noise Reduction Coefficient Rating,
171-72
Noise Tasmania, 34
Noise Watch and Right to Quiet
Society, 34

noisy environment (see *noise, back-ground*)
no-observed adverse effect level,
94-95

O

Obama, President Barrack, 38
occupational exposure (see *noise*)
Occupational Safety and Health
Act, 132-133
Occupational Safety and Health
Administration, 13-14, 33, 45,
50, 132-33, 140, 142
Occupational Safety and Health
Review Comm, 132
Office of Noise Abatement and
Control, 33, 132
Okinawa Prefectual Gov't, 38
Oregon Museum of Sci/Indust, 52-54
organ of Corti, 21-23, 30
ossicles (also see *malleus, incus,
stapes*), 20-21
ossicular chain (see *ossicles*)
otoacoustic emissions, 94
otolaryngologist/otologist, 19, 109,
117-18
otosclerosis, 5
ototoxic meds, 117
ototoxicants (see *chemicals, industrial*)
OurAirspace, 34
outer ear (see *ear*)
oval window, 26

P

Parkinson's disease, 123
partitions (also see *walls*)
high frequency insulator, 174
low frequency insulator, 174
perilymph fluid, 22-23, 93
pharmaceutical drugs, 10
phase cancellation (also see *noise
cancellation*), 71
pitch, 4, 17, 52

pollutants (also see *chemicals, industrial*), 117
potassium, 22, 25
potentiation, 94
presbycusis, 6
pressure (see *sound pressure*)
product liability (see *tort laws*)
propagation, 12

Q

Quiet Communities Act, 33
Quiet Enjoyment, 147
quinine, 117

R

radiotelephony, 90
ratio, signal-to-noise (see *signal-to-noise*)
reactive oxygen species, 98
reading scores, 11
Reagan, Ronald, 33
real-ear attenuation, 156-58
recreational exposure (see *hearing loss; noise*)
Rehab Act, 136
regulating noise (see *noise, reg.*)
Reissner's membrane, 21-23
resonant frequencies, 168,
    defining, 17, 179
reticular lamina, 23
round window, 22, 26
rupture of eardrum (see *eardrum*)

S

Sarbanes-Oxley Act, 142
scala media, 21, 23
scala tympani, 21-23
scala vestibuli, 21-23
scale (see *decibel*)
selenium, 98
sensorineural hearing loss (see *hearing loss, sensorineural*)
signal-to-noise ratio, 86-88
sleep deprivation (see *noise, exp. to*)
sleep disruption, 11

smoking, 117
sodium, 22
sound (also see *absorptive materials*)
    basics of, 11-13
    high frequency, 172
    localizing, 17, 29, 30, 34, 84
    low frequency, 172
    speed of (in),
        air, 2
        steel, 2
        water, 2
    traveling of, 12
sound level meters, 7, 67, 161
sound levels (see *noise*)
    dangerous (see *noise*)
sound pressure levels (SPL), 10-11,
    13-14, 27, 35, 51, 56-61
    defined, 6-9, 12
    directivity of, 165
    distances with, 168-69
    distribution of, 163-180
    reflection of, 166-67
    reverberation, 169-71
    source of, 167
    standing waves in, 167-68
sound transmission, reducing, 171-80
Sound Transmission Class, 174-75, 177
sound waves, 16
speech (also see *consonants; vowels*) 16
spiral ganglion, 28
spiral ligament, 23
standards (see *noise*)
stapes, 20-22,
    footplate of, 26
stereocilia, 24-25
Stewart, Surg Gen William, 37
stirrup (see *stapes*)
stress (see *noise, stress reactions*)
stria vascularis, 21, 23, 25
stroke, 117
Subway Watchdog Comm, 39

superior olivary complex, 29-30
syphilis, 118

T

tectorial membrane, 21, 23
Telecomm Act, 136
Television Decod Circuitry Act, 136
threshold shift,
    permanent, 115
    temporary, 115
threshold (of hearing)
    defining, 3
tinnitus (and hyperacusis), 51-52,
    65-66, 92, 103-13, 117-18,
    137-38
    amygdalae relationship in, 105
    antidepressants and,
        amitriptyline, 120
        nortriptyline, 120
        Paxil, 120
        Prozac, 120
        Valium, 120
        Xanax, 120
        Zoloft, 120
    Bell's palsy and, 118
    cardiovascular effects with, 124
        med eval of, 124-25
        treatment of, 125
    continuous, 117
    defined, 3, 9, 104
    depression with, 118
    earplug use with, 106, 108
    habituation with, 108
    hippocampus with, 105
    insomnia with, 121-22
        causes of, 123
        drug effects with, 123-24
        med eval for, 122-23
        neurological disorders with,
          123
        polysomnogram for, 122
        psychological disorders with,
          123
        treatment for, 123-24
    intermittent, 117

    Lyme disease and, 118
    management of, 119-21
    mechanisms of, 104-106
    medical treatments for, 119-21
    mental health and, 125
    migraine and, 118
    nonpulsatile, 117
    problems with, 106-108
        agitation, 107-108, 110
        anxiety, 103, 105-106, 110
        apprehension, 105, 107
        concentration, 107
        distress, 107-108
        fear, 105-107
        irritability, 103, 105, 108
        isolation, 107
        quality of life, 106
        negative thought, 107
        reduced awareness, 108
        restlessness, 107
        sleep deprivation, 103, 106-
        107
    pulsing, 117
    severity of, 119
    sleep problems with (see *insom-
        nia*)
    sounds with, 108, 110
        intrusive, 108
        painful, 108
        wideband, 110
    suicide and, 138
    therapy (treatment) for, 108-11
        antidepressants (see *tinn,
          antidepress*)
        antihistamine, 120
        biofeedback, 110
        Cognitive Behavioral, 110-
          11, 124
        counseling, 109-10
        drug, 119-21, 123-24
        electrical stim, 108, 119, 121
        habituation-based, 110
        herbal, 120-21
        homeopathy, 119
        laser light, 111

magnetic stim, 108
maskers, 110
mineral, 120
Neuromonics, 110
Pilates, 111
Progressive Audiologic Man-
    agement, 110
relaxation therapy, 110-11
self-help, 111
sound, 110
Tinnitus Retaining, 110-11
TMJ, 118-19, 121
vitamin, 120
vascular abnormalities and, 118
vicious cycle with, 105, 110
tonotopic organization, 28
Toronto Health Dept, 37
Tort Laws, 143
assault, 143
battery, 143
civil claims, 145
criminal claims, 145-47
emotional distress, 143
frivolous complaints re, 145
liability, 143-47
malpractice, 144
negligence, 144-47
Townshend, Pete, 65, 103
toxicants (see *chemicals*)
traffic noise (see *noise*)
transmission loss, 173-80
traveling wave, 26-27
tuberculosis, 92
tuning curves, 28-29
tympanic membrane (see *eardrum*)

U

United Auto Workers, 44
**UK-Heathrow Assn for Control of
    Aircraft Noise,** 34
University of Melbourne, 15
US Constitution, 130
US Court System, 148
US Dept of Health/Human Serv, 133
US Hear Conserv Amendment, 153

US House Comm on Ed and Labor,
    41

V

vacuum cleaners, 13
vertigo, 138
Veterans Administration, 110
vibrations, 2-3, 20, 23, 26, 28, 39,
    77, 155, 173, 178
control of, 178-80
visual cues, 90
vitamins, 98
C, 98
E, 98
von Bekesy, 26
vowels, (also see *frequency*),
    low frequency, 4, 18, 166

W

Walkman®, 61-62
walls (also see *partitions*), 174-76
wax (see *cerumen*)
Whistleblower Protect Act, 142
whistleblowers (see *laws*)
windows, 177
word recognition testing, 5
work interference, 11
Workers' Compensation, 138, 143,
    146
World Health Organization (WHO),
    15, 38, 114, 139-40
Guidelines for Comm Noise
    from, 139
recommended noise levels from,
    149

Other Titles From Auricle Ink Publishers

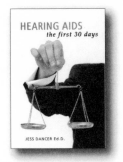

Hearing Aids: the First 30 Days
©2009, Jess Dancer, EdD
Retail $14.95

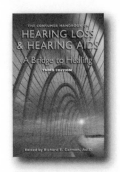

*Consumer Handbook on Hearing Loss
and Hearing Aids* (Third Edition)
©2009, Richard E. Carmen, AuD (Ed)
Retail $18.95/$24.95

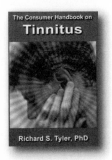

Consumer Handbook on Tinnitus
©2008, Richard S. Tyler, PhD (Ed)
Retail: $32.95

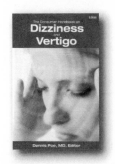

*Consumer Handbook on Dizziness
and Vertigo*
©2005, Dennis Poe, MD (Ed)
Retail: $29.95

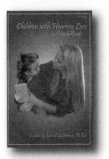

*Children with Hearing Loss
A Family Guide*
©2006, David Luterman, DEd (Ed)
Retail: $16.95

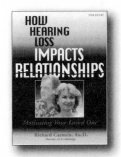

*How Hearing Loss Impacts Relationships
Motivating Your Loved One*
©2005, Richard E. Carmen, AuD
Retail: $15.95

NOTES

NOTES

NOTES

NOTES

NOTES

NOTES

NOTES

NOTES

NOTES

NOTES

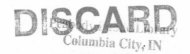